Introduction to Toxicology

Second Edition

D0145684

Introduction to Toxicology

Second Edition

John A. Timbrell
Glaxo Professor of Toxicology
School of Pharmacy
University of London

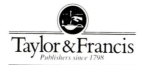

Taylor & Francis
Publishers since 1798

UK   Taylor & Francis Ltd, 4 John Street, London WC1N 2ET

USA   Taylor & Francis Inc., 1900 Frost Road, Suite 101, Bristol, PA 19007

British Library Cataloguing in Publication Data

A catalogue record for this book is available from the British Library
ISBN 0 7484 0240 3 (cloth)
ISBN 0 7484 0241 1 (paper)

Library of Congress Cataloging-in-Publication Data are available

Cover design by OWL Services

Typeset by
Mathematical Composition Setters Ltd, Salisbury, Wiltshire

Printed in Great Britain by Burgess Science Press, Basingstoke on paper which has a specified pH value on final paper manufacture of not less than 7.5 and is therefore 'acid free'.

For
Anna, Becky and Cathy

Contents

Preface to First Edition   xi

Preface to Second Edition   xiii

Chapter 1. Introduction   1
   Historical Aspects   2
   Types of Toxic Substance   6
   Types of Exposure   8
   Dose-Response Relationship   9
   Questions   16
   Bibliography   17

Chapter 2. Disposition of Toxic Compounds   19
   Absorption of Toxic Compounds   19
   Distribution of Toxic Compounds   28
   Excretion of Toxic Compounds   31
   Metabolism of Foreign Compounds   36
   Factors Affecting Toxic Responses   48
   Questions   51
   Bibliography   52

Chapter 3. Types of Exposure and Response   55
   Types of Exposure   55
   Route of Exposure   55
   Types of Toxic Response   56
   Detection of Toxic Responses   60
   Questions   60
   Bibliography   60

Chapter 4. Drugs as Toxic Substances   61
   Introduction   61
   Paracetamol   62
   Hydralazine   63
   Halothane   66

Debrisoquine 67
Thalidomide 69
Drug Interactions 69
Altered Responsiveness: Glucose-6-phosphate Dehydrogenase
Deficiency 70
Questions 71
Bibliography 71

Chapter 5. Industrial Chemicals 73
Industrial Chemicals 73
Means of Exposure 73
Toxic Effects 74
Vinyl Chloride 75
Cadmium 76
Aromatic Amines 77
Asbestos 78
Legislation 80
Question 81
Bibliography 81

Chapter 6. Food Additives and Contaminants 83
Introduction 83
Tartrazine 85
Saccharin 86
Food Contaminants 87
The Spanish Oil Syndrome 88
Questions 89
Bibliography 90

Chapter 7. Pesticides 91
Introduction 91
DDT 92
Organophosphorus Compounds 96
Paraquat 97
Fluoroacetate 100
Questions 100
Bibliography 101

Chapter 8. Environmental Pollutants 103
Introduction 103
Air Pollution 104
Particulates 107
Acid Rain 108
Lead Pollution 111
Water Pollution 114
Food Chains 115
Mercury and Methylmercury 118

Questions 121
Bibliography 121

Chapter 9. Natural Products 123
Plant Toxins 123
Animal Toxins 125
Fungal Toxins 128
Microbial Toxins 129
Question 129
Bibliography 129

Chapter 10. Household Products 131
Introduction 131
Carbon Monoxide 133
Antifreeze: Ethylene Glycol 135
Alcohol 136
Glue Sniffing and Solvent Abuse 137
Questions 137
Bibliography 137

Chapter 11. Toxicity Testing and Risk Assessment 139
Introduction 139
Acute Toxicity Tests 141
Sub-acute Toxicity Tests 142
Chronic Toxicity Tests 143
Risk Assessment and Interpretation of Toxicological Data 145
Conclusions 149
Questions 149
Bibliography 149

Glossary 151

Index 161

Preface to First Edition

There is an ever increasing use of chemicals in modern society and, because of this, toxicology is becoming an increasingly important subject. Taught courses are now available in different countries at various levels to educate young toxicologists. Currently, however, there are no introductory texts that are reasonably inexpensive, and that serve as an introduction to the subject for students with backgrounds in various disciplines. Thus, there are hardback textbooks, such as *Cassarett and Doull's Toxicology*, for dedicated toxicologists and various specialist texts for particular aspects of toxicology. The smaller textbooks that are available are generally biased towards one particular aspect or interpretation of toxicology, such as the biochemical, pathological, pharmacological or pharmacokinetic aspects. However, most of these are either too expensive or too specialist for the novice toxicologist, the undergraduate or the postgraduate who simply wishes to become familiar with the subject as a whole.

Toxicology is a multidisciplinary subject, which has a large and diffuse literature and it is developing rapidly. Bringing this information together is difficult and time consuming for the student. Consequently there is a need for a cohesive text at the introductory rather than more advanced level. These deficiencies in the market became clear to me whilst being involved in teaching first a Masters course and then a Bachelors degree course in toxicology.

This book, therefore, has arisen from my awareness of the need for an introductory text for myself and for my own students and its content is largely based upon the information I have amassed in the preparation of lectures for these same students. I am indebted to these students for being the foil for this preparation and also to various colleagues for their helpful comments.

London, 1988

Preface to Second Edition

Since the first edition of this book, toxicology has become a more mature science and has advanced in a number of ways, especially at the basic mechanistic level. However, the basic principles of the science have remained largely unchanged. Therefore the revision has not been a major one.

The purpose of this book was to be an introductory text for beginners rather than an encyclopedic toxicology text or a specialist mechanistic monograph. Consequently the revision has been mainly concerned with adding new details to the examples previously used, adding some new examples and updating certain points. The bibliography has however been extensively revised. Also, questions have now been added for use both by teachers and students. More toxicology texts have appeared on the market since the first edition of this book, but these have all been either specialist or relatively large as was previously the case. *Cassarett and Doull's Toxicology* is still available (now in a 4th edition) for dedicated toxicologists and other similar texts have been published. However, these are either too expensive or specialist for the novice toxicologist or scientist who simply wants an overview in order to become familiar with the subject as a whole. Therefore, there is still a need for an introductory text. There are now many more courses and course units in toxicology reflecting greater awareness of the subject and, hence, the need for an introductory text is, if anything, greater than before. I hope this revised edition caters for this need.

I am grateful to all those who have helped directly and indirectly in the preparation of this edition and those who helped in the preparation of the first edition are duly acknowledged in the preface to that edition. Thanks in particular to Mary Fagg for the final preparations to the manuscript and to Gerry Kenna for the information on halothane. Special thanks go to my family for their tolerance and support.

London, July 1994

Chapter 1

Introduction

Toxicology is the study of the harmful interactions between chemicals and biological systems. Man, the other animals, and the plants in the modern world are increasingly being exposed to chemicals of an enormous variety. These chemicals range from metals and inorganic chemicals to large complex organic molecules, yet they are all potentially toxic. The study of the pathological, biochemical and physiological effects of such substances is the fascinating brief of the toxicologist. Toxicology, like medicine, is a multidisciplinary subject which encompasses many areas. This makes it an absorbing and challenging area of research. The challenge of toxicology is to apply basic biochemical, chemical, pathological and physiological knowledge along with experimental observation to gain an understanding of why certain substances cause the disruption in a biological system which may lead to toxic effects.

Approximately 65 000 chemicals are currently produced in the USA and 500–1000 new chemicals are added each year. Because of this escalation in the numbers of chemicals to which our environment may be exposed (Figure 1.1), it has become increasingly important to have some knowledge of the toxic effects they may have and to attempt to measure and assess these effects.

In recent years, awareness of the problem of human and animal exposure to potentially toxic chemicals in our environment has grown. Perhaps one of the first to bring this to the attention of the public was Rachel Carson with her book *Silent Spring*. This was a description of the devastating effects of pesticides on the flora and fauna of the North American environment. As discussed by Efron in her book *The Apocalyptics, Cancer and the Big Lie* (1984), Carson and certain later scientists probably exaggerated the dangers of chemicals, but her message was quite clear. Few would disagree that man should beware of the synthetic chemicals to which the environment is exposed. Thus, toxicology has another dimension: the social, moral and legal aspects of exposure of populations to chemicals of unknown or uncertain hazard. Hazard and risk assessments and value judgements become important. The toxicologist is often asked to make such assessments and judgements. So toxicology has a very important role to play in modern society and consequently it is now growing rapidly as a new subject.

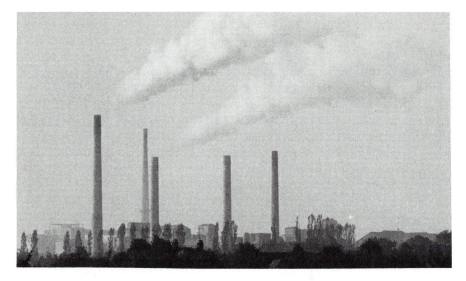

Figure 1.1. Toxicology is concerned with the exposure of living systems in the environment to toxic substances from a variety of sources.

Historical Aspects

Toxicology has been called the study of poisons, but this poses the question 'what is a poison?' Poisons can range from a naturally occurring plant alkaloid to a synthetic nerve gas. A poison is any substance which has a harmful effect on a living system; whether we regard a substance as a poison or not may depend on its use. For example, humans can protect themselves against the effects of harmful bacteria by killing them with antibiotics, such as penicillin; alternatively, humans can kill each other with the war gas phosgene. Both phosgene and penicillin, therefore, are poisons in the strictest sense of the word but we regard them entirely differently.

It is only recently that the study of poisons has become a truly scientific pursuit. In the past it was mainly a practical art utilized by murderers and assassins. Poison, as a subtle and silent weapon, has played an important part in human history.

Primitive man was aware of natural poisons from animals and plants and indeed used these on his weapons. The word toxicology is derived from *toxicon* – a poisonous substance into which arrow heads were dipped and *toxikos* – a bow. The study of poisons must have started by 1500 BC because the Ebers Papyrus, the earliest collection of medical records, contains many references and recipes for poisons. The ancient Egyptians were able to distil prussic acid from peach kernels, poisons such as arsenic, aconite and opium were also known to Hindu medicine as recorded in the Vedas, around 900 BC and the ancient Chinese used aconite as an arrow poison. Hippocrates in his writings (400 BC) showed that the ancient Greeks had a professional awareness of poisons and of the principles of toxicology, particularly with regard to the treatment of poisoning by influencing absorption. Poisoning was relatively common in ancient Greece so the study of poisons and the development of antidotes in particular was important. For example, Nicander of Colophon, (185–135 BC) physician to Attalus, King of Bythnia, was allowed to experiment with poisons using condemned criminals as subjects. As a result of his studies he wrote a treatise on antidotes to poisonous reptiles and substances (Theriaca and Alexipharmica) and mentioned 22 specific poisons including ceruse (white lead), litharge (lead oxide), aconite (wolfsbane), cantharides, conium (hemlock), hyoscyamus (henbane) and opium. He recommended linseed tea to induce vomiting and sucking the venom from the bite of a venomous animal as treatments. Similarly, King Mithridates used criminals to search for antidotes to venom and poisonous substances and regularly protected himself with a mixture of 50 different antidotes (Mithridatum). Legend has it that he was unable to poison himself when suicide became necessary! The term mithridatic (meaning antidote) is derived from his name.

The first known law against poisoning was issued in Rome by Sulla in 82 BC to protect against careless dispensing. The Greek physician Dioscorides (AD 50) made a particularly significant contribution to toxicology by classifying poisons as animal, plant or mineral and recognizing the value of emetics in the treatment of poisoning. His treatise on Materia Medica was the major work on poisons for fifteen centuries.

So, the origins of toxicology lie in the use of poisons for murder, suicide and political assassination. It is well known for example that Socrates committed suicide by taking hemlock (Figure 1.2). There are many examples of poisons being used for nefarious purposes such as the poisoning of Claudius and his son Britannicus with arsenic. In the latter case, Nero employed a professional poisoner who put the arsenic into the water used to cool the soup and so avoided the taster. The prolific use of poisons in this way made it necessary for treatments to be devised and Maimmonides (1135–1204) wrote *Poisons and Their Antidotes* which detailed some of the treatments thought to be effective.

In the Middle Ages, especially in Italy, the art of poisoning for political ends developed into a cult. The Borgias were infamous during the fifteenth and sixteenth centuries. In seventeenth-century Italy, a woman by the name of Toffana prepared cosmetics containing arsenic (Aqua Toffana) which were used to remove unwanted rivals, husbands and enemies! Similarly Catherine de Medici prepared poisons and tested them on the poor and sick of France, noting all the clinical signs and symptoms.

One of the most significant historic figures in the development of the science of toxicology is Paracelsus (1493–1541) who saw the need for proper experimentation and gave the subject a scientific basis. He distinguished between the therapeutic and toxic properties of substances and recognized that these may be indistinguishable except by dose, giving rise to the concept of the dose-response relationship. Another significant figure in toxicology was Orfila, a Spanish physician (1787–1853) who recognized it as a separate discipline and contributed to forensic toxicology by devising means of detecting poisonous substances and therefore proving that poisoning had taken place. From then

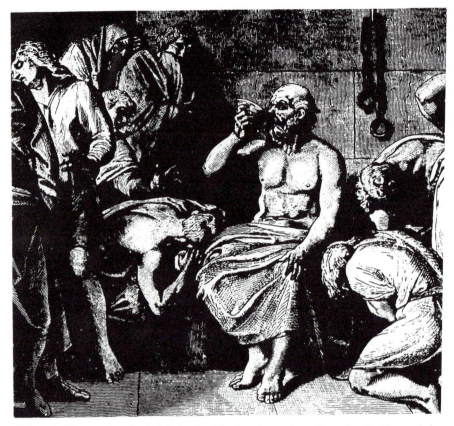

Figure 1.2. Socrates drinking hemlock, the Athenian state poison. Reproduced with permission from the Mary Evans Picture Library, London.

on toxicology began to develop in a more scientific manner and began to include the study of the mechanism of action of poisons. Indeed Claude Bernard (1813–1878) believed that the study of the effects of substances on biological systems could enhance the understanding of those systems. He identified the site of action of curare as either the nerve ending or the neuro-muscular junction.

More recently, Sir Rudolph Peters studied the mechanism of action of arsenical war gases and so devised the effective antidote known as British Anti-Lewisite in 1945. Other examples include cyanide, which is an inhibitor of oxidative phosphorylation, and fluorocitrate, which is a specific inhibitor of aconitase, one of the enzymes involved in the Krebs cycle. Both compounds have been used experimentally to aid in the understanding of normal bio-chemical processes.

Toxicology has now become much more than the use of poisons for nefarious purposes and the production of antidotes to them. The enormous and ever increasing number (65 000+) of man-made chemicals in the environment to which we may potentially be exposed has thrust toxicology into the limelight.

It has also created the need for the organized study of toxic substances by the industries manufacturing them and for legislation to control them. This has in turn resulted in the establishment of government regulatory agencies to implement the resulting legislation.

Some of the industrial disasters which have occurred in recent times have highlighted the need for knowledge of the toxicity of compounds used in industry as well as for drugs and food additives. This knowledge is essential for the development of effective and rapid treatment of the toxic effects, just as it is essential for the treatment of overdoses and accidental poisonings. For example, one of the worst industrial disasters occurred at Bhopal in India in 1984 where a factory manufacturing the insecticide carbaryl leaked a large amount of the extremely noxious compound methyl isocyanate (Figure 1.3). Little was known of the toxicity of this compound and consequently treatment of the victims was uncertain and possibly inadequate.

Another major reason for testing chemicals in toxicity and other studies is so that they may be classified according to hazard such as toxic, explosive or flammable. This will then enable decisions to be made about marketing and labelling. So we are exposed to toxic or potentially toxic compounds in many ways in our daily lives and toxicology is clearly a subject of great importance in society. This becomes apparent when we look at the types of poisons and the ways in which we are exposed to them. Indeed, the categories cover virtually all the chemicals one might expect to encounter in the environment. After consideration of this one might well ask 'are all chemicals toxic?' The following phrase perhaps provides an answer: 'there are no safe chemicals, only safe ways of using them.'

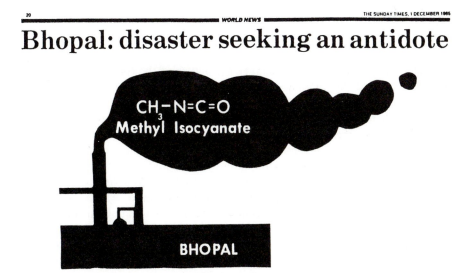

Figure 1.3. A headline reminds us that a year after the disaster in Bhopal, India, in which thousands were killed and injured by the toxic chemical methyl isocyanate accidentally released from a chemical plant, there is no cure or antidote.
Headline from *The Sunday Times*, 1 December 1985, with permission.

Types of Toxic Substance

Toxic substances fall into several classes in relation to the way man is exposed
to them: drugs, food additives, pesticides, industrial chemicals, environmental
pollutants, natural toxins and household poisons. Each of these categories will
be discussed in more detail in later chapters but they will be briefly introduced
here.

Drugs

Most people in the Western world consume drugs of one sort or another
throughout their lives. Drugs, however, have usually been designed to be
highly potent in biological systems and consequently many are potentially
toxic. Drug toxicity may be due either to an overdose or it may be a rare and
unusual adverse effect, and examples of both of these will be considered in
detail in Chapter 4.

Drugs vary enormously in chemical structure and possess a wide variety of
biological activities. They are probably the only foreign substances of known
biological activity that man ingests intentionally. Included in this category are
alcohol and the active principles in cigarettes, both of which are used because
of their biological activity and both, of course, have toxic properties. Drugs
used in veterinary practice must also be considered here (and in the next
section) as humans may consume meat from or other food derived from
animals treated with these drugs.

Food Additives

This is the second category of foreign substances which are directly ingested.
However, food additives are usually of low biological activity. Many different
additives are now added to food to alter the flavour or colour, prevent
spoilage, or in some other way change the nature of the foodstuff. There are
also many potentially toxic substances which may be regarded as contaminants
occurring naturally in food, resulting from cooking, or from other contamination, and specific examples will be discussed in a later chapter. Veterinary
drugs and their breakdown products may also be found in foodstuffs as
indicated above. Most of these substances, both natural and artificial, may be
present in food in very small amounts but for the majority little is known of
their long-term toxicity. In many cases they are ingested daily for perhaps a
lifetime and the numbers of people exposed is very large. Although reliable
data is still scarce, there certainly seems to be evidence that at least some additives may be associated with adverse effects. Public awareness of this has now
begun to influence the preparation and manufacture of food such that additive
free foods are appearing on supermarket shelves.

Industrial Chemicals

Industrial chemicals may contribute to environmental pollution (considered next), and they may be a direct hazard in the workplace where they are used, formulated or manufactured. There is a huge range of chemical types and many different industries may involve the use or manufacture of hazardous chemicals. In the broadest sense industrial exposure might include exposure to the solvents used in photocopiers and typists' correction fluid. Although in general exposure is controlled by law, often by the setting of control limits, realistic levels may still prove to be hazardous in the long term and acute exposure due to accidents will always occur. The long development time of diseases such as cancer often makes it difficult to determine the cause until sufficient of the workforce have presented with the disease for the association with the toxic compound to be made.

Environmental Pollutants

The main sources of pollution are industrial processes and the deliberate release into the environment of substances such as pesticides. The most visible pollutant, but perhaps not the most significant is smoke from power stations and factories. Factories may also produce and emit more potent substances in smaller quantities although the level of these is generally controlled. Environmental pollutants may be released into the air, river or sea water or dumped onto land. Car exhaust fumes with several known toxic constituents constitute a major source of pollution.

Pesticides are deliberately sprayed onto crops or agricultural land with the potential for exposure either via the crop itself or through contamination of drinking water or air. With pesticides a major problem is persistence in the environment and an increase in concentration during passage through the food chain.

Natural Toxins

Many plants and animals produce toxic substances for both defensive and offensive purposes. Natural toxins of animal, plant and bacterial origin comprise a wide variety of chemical types, cause a variety of toxic effects and are a significant cause of human poisonings. The concept currently expounded by some individuals that 'natural is safe' is in many cases very far from the truth and some of the most toxic substances known to man are of natural origin. Natural toxins may feature in poisoning via contamination in food, by accidental ingestion of poisonous plants or animals, and by stinging and biting.

Household Poisons

These may include some of the substances in the other categories such as pesticides, drugs and solvents. Exposure to these types of compounds is usually acute rather than chronic. Many of the household substances used for cleaning are irritants and some are corrosive. Consequently, they may cause severe skin and eye lesions to humans if they are exposed. If swallowed in significant quantities or if highly concentrated solutions are ingested, some household materials such as bleach and caustic soda can cause severe tissue damage to the oesophagus and stomach. Some of the drugs and pesticides which are widely available and consequently often found in the home are also very toxic. For example, the herbicide paraquat and the drug paracetamol are both toxic and have both contributed significantly to human poisoning deaths.

Types of Exposure

In some cases the means of exposure is determined by the nature of the toxic substance. For example, gases and vapours lead to inhalation exposure whereas liquids give rise to problems associated with skin contact. Many industrial chemicals are often associated with chronic effects due to long term exposure whereas household substances are usually involved in acute poisoning following a single episode of accidental exposure.

The types of exposure will be briefly discussed at this introductory stage but will be discussed again more fully in later chapters.

Intentional Ingestion

Drugs and food additives are taken in by many millions of people every day, in some cases for long periods of time. The exposure to these compounds, especially repeated or chronic exposure may be associated with adverse responses such as allergic reactions. Alcohol and cigarettes are used by many people, often on a long-term basis, and these may lead to chronic toxic effects.

Occupational Exposure

Occupational exposure to toxic compounds is mainly chronic, continual exposure. The route of exposure is either via inhalation or skin contact. Consequently lung disease and dermatitis are common industrial diseases. Acute exposure may occur in the event of an accident such as an explosion, spillage or leakage or because of bad working practices. Cleaning out reactor vessels which have contained solvents may lead to acute toxicity due to excessive exposure for example.

Environmental Exposure

Effluents from factories, either gaseous or liquid may sometimes briefly, or more often continuously, contaminate our immediate environment and also more distant environments such as the seas and oceans or the atmosphere in other countries. This form of exposure is usually chronic but there have been isolated accidents at factories where acute exposure of humans outside the factory occurs such as at Bhopal and Seveso. Chronic exposure to gases such as sulphur dioxide, nitrogen oxides and carbon monoxide occurs in industrial areas and regions of heavy traffic and may cause acute irritation but the chronic toxic effects are largely unknown.

Environmental exposure is also important in relation to pesticides contaminating air, water and food. Large scale spraying means that most people are exposed to pesticides or their residues both within their food and directly via the air.

Accidental Poisoning

This type of exposure is usually acute rather than chronic. Drugs, pesticides, household products and natural poisons may all be involved in this type of exposure, and children and the elderly are most commonly involved. Mistaken ingestion of a poisonous plant, cleaning fluid or drug falls into this category as does accidental ingestion of an excessive dose of a drug. Inhalation of fumes from fires and stoves is also an important cause of accidental poisoning.

Intentional Poisoning

Fortunately homicide by poisoning is now relatively rare but suicide by poisoning is regrettably all too common. Drugs are commonly used but household products occasionally feature; both types are usually taken by mouth in these circumstances.

Dose-Response Relationship

'All substances are poisons; there is none which is not a poison. The right dose differentiates a poison and a remedy' Paracelsus (1493-1541).

Paracelsus was probably the first to recognize the concept that toxicity is a relative phenomenon and that it depends not only on the toxic properties but on the dose of the compound administered. This relationship between the dose of a compound and the response it elicits is a fundamental concept in toxicology. However, first we must consider the nature of the response itself. The toxic response that is simplest to observe is death but this is a crude parameter to measure. Another indicator of a toxic response is the presence of a pathological lesion such as liver cell necrosis. A more precisely measured response is a biochemical, pharmacological or chemical change.

We can distinguish between so-called 'all or none' responses, such as death, and graded responses, such as the inhibition of an enzyme or the level of a marker of pathological damage. Both 'all or none' responses and graded responses can show a typical dose response relation. In both cases there will be a dose at which there is no measurable effect and an upper dose where there is a maximal response. Very often in a toxicity study, either in whole animals or in isolated cells, lethality will be the first parameter of toxicity utilized but this gives little if any information about the underlying mechanism of toxicity. However, it is often important to know the limits of dosing in practical terms.

Although it is not always necessary to know the lethal dose, it is important to know whether toxicity occurs at the dose or a multiple of the dose likely to be encountered by man or animals. However in certain situations it is extremely difficult or impossible to quantify the likely human dose and may be similarly difficult to extrapolate the likely effects in man from the available data (see also Chapter 11).

It should be noted that strictly speaking the word dose means the total amount of a substance administered to an organism whereas the term dosage includes a characteristic of the organism, typically body weight or surface area. Dosage is more precise, therefore, and can be related to other organisms, for example as mg substance/kg body weight. We can therefore talk about dosage-response relationships.

With 'all or none' responses (lethality for example) the normal way to determine and represent the dose response relation is to determine the percentage of the animals or cells in a particular dosage or concentration group which show the response. This response is then plotted against the dosage or concentration resulting in a typical sigmoid curve as illustrated in Figure 1.4. By using probit analysis the data can be plotted as a straight line (Figures 1.5 and 1.6).

When the response is a graded one the actual values measured are plotted against the dosage or concentration giving the same type of curve (Figure 1.4).

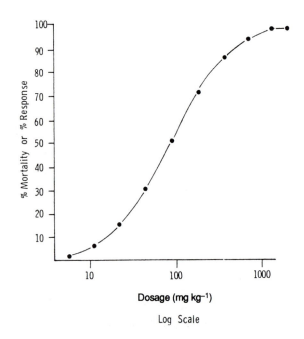

Figure 1.4. A typical dose-response curve where the percentage response or mortality is plotted against the log of the dosage.
From Timbrell, J. A., *Principles of Biochemical Toxicology*, Taylor & Francis, London, 1991.

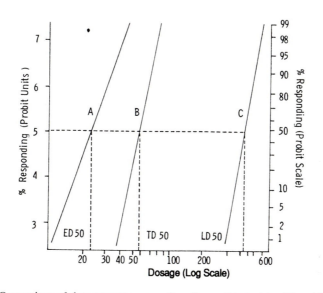

Figure 1.5. Comparison of dose-response curves for efficacy (A), toxicity (B) and lethality (C). The effective, toxic or lethal dosage for 50% of the animals in the group can be estimated as shown. This graph shows the relationship between these parameters. The proximity of the ED_{50} and TD_{50} indicates the margin of safety of the compound. (Probits are units of standard deviation, where the median is probit 5).
From Timbrell, J. A., *Principles of Biochemical Toxicology*, Taylor & Francis, London, 1991.

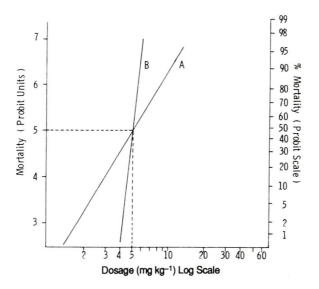

Figure 1.6. Comparison of the toxicity of two compounds A and B. Although they both have the same LD_{50} (or TD_{50}) compound A is more *potent* than compound B.
From Timbrell, J. A., *Principles of Biochemical Toxicology*, Taylor & Francis, London, 1991.

Receptors

In some cases toxic effects are due to the interaction between the compound and a specific molecular receptor site. This receptor might be an enzyme which could be inhibited, or some other macromolecule, but in many cases its identity is unknown. Two examples where the receptor is known are carbon monoxide, which interacts specifically with haemoglobin (see Chapter 10), and cyanide, which interacts specifically with the enzyme cytochrome a_3 of the electron transport chain. The toxic effects of these two compounds are a direct result of these interactions and, it is assumed, depend on the number of molecules of the toxic compound bound to the receptors. Thus, the more molecules of the receptor that are occupied by the toxic compound the greater the toxic effect. There will be a concentration of the toxic compound at which all of the molecules of the receptor are occupied, however, and hence there will be no further increase in the toxic effect. This relationship gives rise to the classical dose response curve (Figure 1.4). It is beyond the scope of this book to discuss this in more detail but several of the references in the bibliography may be consulted for more information.

Therefore the interpretation of the dose response relationship is based on certain assumptions:

1. the response is proportional to the concentration at the target site;
2. the concentration at the target site is related to the dose;
3. the response is causally related to the compound administered.

The target site might be a receptor in which case the dose-response relationship may be similar to those observed with pharmacological effects. That is the receptor must be occupied by the toxic compound in order for there to be a response and there will be a point at which all the receptors are occupied, giving the maximum response.

However, unlike the situation in pharmacology the study of receptors has not yet featured prominently in toxicology and there are few examples where specific receptors are known to be directly involved in the mediation of toxic effects. The two examples given above are fairly straightforward cases and there are some other similar examples of enzyme inhibition. However, with some toxic effects such as the production of liver necrosis caused by paracetamol for instance, although a dose-response relation can be demonstrated there may be no simple toxicant-receptor interaction in the classical sense. Although a toxic response may be observed after exposure to a substance at one particular dose, it is usual to demonstrate responses at several doses of the compound in question and that there is a relationship between the dose and the magnitude of the response.

The shape of the dose-response curve depends on the type of toxic effect measured and the mechanism underlying it. For example, when cyanide reacts with cytochrome a_3 it binds irreversibly and curtails the function of the electron transport chain in the mitochondria. As this is a function vital to the life of the cell the dose-response curve for lethality is very steep for cyanide.

The more precise the measurement made and the greater the number of determinations the more precise will be the curve and parameters derived from it.

Once a dose-response relationship has been demonstrated there are several parameters which can be derived from it. When lethality has been used as an endpoint, the LD_{50} can be determined (Figure 1.5). This is defined as the dosage of a substance which kills 50 per cent of the animals in a particular group, usually determined in an acute, single exposure study. It is not an exact value and in recent years there has been much discussion as to its usefulness and necessity in toxicology (see Chapter 11). The LD_{50} value may vary for the same compound between different groups of the same species of animal. The value itself is only of real use in a comparative sense, giving the toxicologist an idea of how toxic a compound is relative to other substances (Table 1.1, Figure 1.6) or enabling toxicity to be compared using various routes of administration (Table 1.2) or in different species for example (Table 1.3). It is also widely used for classification purposes, such as hazard warnings for example. Recently there has been a proposal by the British Toxicology Society for an alternative means of assessing the relative harmfulness of a compound which simply involves dosing a few animals with a range of doses and noting the responses. The chemical can then be classified as for example very toxic, toxic or not very toxic without the use of the LD_{50} test. (For a further discussion see Chapter 11.)

Table 1.1 Approximate LD_{50} values for a variety of chemical substances

Compound	LD_{50} mg kg^{-1}
Ethanol	10,000
DDT	100
Nicotine	1
Tetrodotoxin	0.1
Dioxin	0.001
Botulinus toxin	0.00001

Source: T. A. Loomis (1974), *Essentials of Toxicology*, 2nd ed. (Philadelphia: Lea & Febiger).

Table 1.2 Effect of route of administration on the toxicity of various compounds.

Route of administration	Pentobarbital[1] LD_{50} mg kg^{-1}	Isoniazid[1] LD_{50} mg kg^{-1}	Procaine[1] LD_{50} mg kg^{-1}	DFP[2] LD_{50} mg kg^{-1}
Oral	280	142	500	4.0
Subcutaneous	130	160	800	1.0
Intramuscular	124	140	630	0.9
Intraperitoneal	130	132	230	1.0
Intravenous	80	153	45	0.3

[1] Mouse toxicity data.
[2] Di-isopropylfluoro phosphate; Rabbit toxicity data.
Source: T. A. Loomis (1968), *Essentials of Toxicology* (Philadelphia: Lea & Febiger).

Table 1.3. Species differences in toxicity of ipomeanol.

	LD_{50} mg kg^{-1}*	Location of tissue damage		
		Liver	Kidney	Lung
Rabbit (New Zealand White)	40	-	-	+
Mouse (A/J Strain)	20	-	+	+
Rat (Fisher Strain)	12	-	-	+
Hamster (Syrian Golden)	140	+	-	+
Guinea Pig (Hartley)	30	-	-	+

* The ipomeanol was administered intraperitoneally in 25% aqueous propylene glycol to all species.
Source: J. S. Dutcher and M. R. Boyd (1979), *Biochem. Pharmacol.* **28**, 3367.

The ED_{50} (effective dosage for 50 per cent) and the TD_{50} (toxic dosage for 50 per cent) are similar parameters to the LD_{50} (Figure 1.5). They can be derived from the dose-response curve where the pharmacological effect or the toxic effect is plotted against dosage instead of lethality. The response can be measured either as the proportion of the group responding (quantal) or as the actual effect, such as blockade of a receptor or degree of pathological damage.

Comparison of the LD_{50} or TD_{50} with the ED_{50} affords an indication of the margin of safety of the compound and it is quantified as the therapeutic index:

$$\frac{LD_{50}}{ED_{50}} \text{ or } \frac{TD_{50}}{ED_{50}}$$

The larger the number the greater is the margin of safety for use of the compound.

Comparison of the curves directly will give the same information (Figure 1.5) and comparison of dose response curves for different compounds will indicate which is the more hazardous (Figure 1.6).

Exposure to toxic compounds sometimes involves mixtures of two or more substances. The effects of such mixtures may be different from the effects of each constituent separately and consequently may be unpredictable. The simplest situation is when each compound has similar effects and the overall toxicity of the mixture is the sum of the individual toxic effects. The effects are then described as additive. However, this may not necessarily be the case; for example, two substances may cause a greater response together than the sum of the individual responses. This is known as a synergistic effect. For example, carbon tetrachloride and alcohol together are more toxic to the liver than expected from the sum of the two individual toxic effects. Potentiation is a similar effect except that the two compounds in question may have different toxic effects or only one may be toxic. For example, the drug disulphiram (antabuse) at non-toxic doses potentiates the toxicity of alcohol and is used for the treatment of alcohol abuse. The drug inhibits the enzyme aldehyde dehydrogenase and so allows an accumulation of acetaldehyde (ethanal) which has unpleasant effects.

The converse effect sometimes observed is a decreased response from a mixture compared with the constituents. This is referred to as antagonism. After repeated exposure, the response may lessen despite similar dosage; tolerance has developed. This may be due to induction of enzymes (see Chapter 2) and hence increased metabolism or to a change in the response or number of receptors. Alternatively repeated exposure can result in accumulation and an exaggerated response.

Such effects must of course be considered when assessing risk from exposure to chemicals and attempting to predict effects.

The Threshold Dose and No Observed Adverse Effect Level (NOAEL)

For some compounds and types of toxic effect there will clearly be a dose below which no effect or response is measurable. There is thus a threshold dose. This can be clearly demonstrated for quantal responses such as lethality, the presence or absence of a pathological lesion or a teratogenic effect for example. This means that there will be a dose at which the response does not occur in any individuals in the population (Figure 1.7). Alternatively the concept could apply to a variable response such as enzyme inhibition which can be measured with increasing concentrations of the compound in question.

The concept of a threshold dose for the toxic effect is an important one in toxicology because it implies that there is a 'no observed adverse effect level', or NOAEL. While this is generally accepted for most types of toxic effect, for chemical carcinogenesis mediated via a genotoxic mechanism this is a controversial issue. In the case of such carcinogens the dose-response curve when extrapolated seems to cross the x-axis at the origin rather than at some positive value or dosage level (Figure 1.7). This means that there is a response at all exposure levels tested and so within the limits of the analytical techniques available no safe exposure level can be set with confidence.

The NOAEL is important for setting exposure limits. For example, the acceptable daily intake (ADI) is based on the NOAEL. This is a factor used to determine the safe intake for food additives and contaminants such as pesticides and residues of veterinary drugs and, hence, to establish the safe level in food. The ADI is determined by the use of a suitable safety factor which may be any factor up to 1000, but is usually 100:

$$ADI = \frac{NOAEL \text{ mg kg}^{-1} \text{ day}^{-1}}{100}$$

In the industrial setting, exposure is regulated in a similar way and the term used is the Threshold Limit Value (TLV;USA) or Maximum Exposure Limit (MEL, UK) which is usually based on exposure for an eight-hour working day (see also Chapters 5 and 11). The NOAEL is usually based on animal toxicity

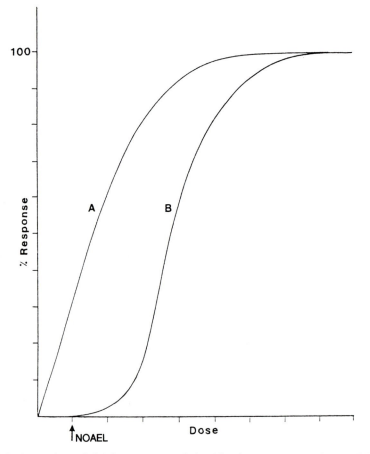

Figure 1.7. Comparison of the dose-response relationships for two compounds A and B. For compound A there is a response at any dose with no threshold. For compound B there is a dose or threshold level below which there is No Observed Adverse Effect (NOAEL). For compounds such as A there is no safe dose.

studies with the compound in question, using the most sensitive species and most discriminating test.

It is clear therefore that the dose-response relationship is a crucial concept in toxicology.

Questions

1. Discuss the dose response relationship and illustrate why it is important in toxicology.
2. Define the terms NOAEL and Therapeutic Index. Explain how a knowledge of these is used in the assessment of toxicological data.

3. Write short notes on the following in relation to toxicology:

   (a) methyl isocyanate;
   (b) Paracelsus;
   (c) LD_{50};
   (d) cyanide;
   (e) synergism.

Bibliography

Albert, A. (1979) *Selective Toxicity*, London: Chapman & Hall.

Albert, A. (1987) *Xenobiosis*, London: Chapman & Hall.

Anderson, D. and Conning, D. M. (Eds) (1988) *Experimental Toxicology. The Basic Principles*, Cambridge: Royal Society of Chemistry.

Ballantyne, B., Marrs, T. and Turner, P. (Eds) (1993) *General and Applied Toxicology*, Basingstoke, UK: Macmillan.

Brown, V. K. (1988) *Acute and Sub-acute Toxicology*, London: Edward Arnold.

Carson, R. (1965) *Silent Spring*, London: Chapman & Hall.

Cassarett and Doull's Toxicology, Amdur, M. O., Doull, J. and Klaassen, C. (Eds) (1991) 4th edition, New York: Pergamon Press.

Deichmann, W. B., Henschler, D., Holmstedt, B. and Keil, G. (1986) What is there that is not a poison: a study of the Third Defense by Paracelsus, *Archives of Toxicology*, **58**, 207.

Efron, E. (1984) *The Apocalyptics, Cancer and the Big Lie*, New York: Simon & Shuster.

Hayes, A. W. (Ed.) (1989) *Principles and Methods of Toxicology*, 2nd edition, New York: Raven Press.

Hodgson, E. and Levi, P. E. (1987) *A Textbook of Modern Toxicology*, Barking: Elsevier.

Lu, F. C. (1991) *Basic Toxicology*, 2nd edition, Washington DC: Hemisphere.

Mann, J. (1994) *Murder, Magic and Medicine*, Oxford: Oxford University Press.

McClellan, R. O. (Ed.) (1971) *Critical Reviews in Toxicology*, Boca Raton, Florida: CRC Press.

Moriarty, F. (1988) *Ecotoxicology: The Study of Pollutants in Ecosystems*, 2nd edition, London: Academic Press.

Munter, S. (Ed.), (1966) *Treatise on Poisons and Their Antidotes*, vol. II of the Medical Writings of Moses Maimonides, Philadelphia: J. P. Lippincott.

Thompson, C. J. S. (1931) *Poisons and Poisoners*, London: H. Shaylor.

Timbrell, J. A. (1991) *Principles of Biochemical Toxicology*, 2nd edition, London: Taylor & Francis.

Volans, G. N., Sims, J., Sullivan, F. M. and Turner, P. (Eds) (1990) *Basic Science in Toxicology*, Proceedings of the Vth International Congress of Toxicology, London: Taylor & Francis.

World Health Organisation (1978) *Principles and Methods for Evaluating the Toxicity of Chemicals. Part I. Environmental Health Criteria 6* Geneva: WHO.

Zbinden, G. (1988) Biopharmaceutical studies, a key to better toxicology, *Xenobiotica*, **18**, suppl. 1, 9.

Chapter 2

Disposition of Toxic Compounds

The disposition of a toxic compound in a biological system may be divided into four phases: absorption, distribution, metabolism and excretion. These four phases are interrelated:

$$\text{Absorption} \rightarrow \text{Distribution} \rightarrow \text{Metabolism}$$
$$\searrow \qquad \qquad \swarrow$$
$$\text{Excretion}$$

and we shall consider each of them in turn.

Absorption of Toxic Compounds

Before a substance can exert a toxic effect it must come into contact with a biological system. Indeed the means, the rate and the site of absorption may all be important factors in the eventual toxicity of a compound. There are several sites for first contact between a toxic compound and a biological system but absorption necessarily involves the passage across cell membranes whichever site is involved. Consequently it is important to consider first the structure and characteristics of biological membranes in order to understand the passage of substances across them.

Membranes are composed mainly of phospholipids and proteins with the lipids arranged as a bilayer interspersed with proteins as shown in Figure 2.1. The particular proteins and phospholipids incorporated into the membrane vary depending on the cell type in which the membrane is located. The proteins may be structural or have a specific function, such as a carrier for membrane transport. The phospholipids may have one of several polar head groups (Figure 2.2) and the fatty acid chains may be saturated, unsaturated or a mixture of both. The degree of saturation will influence the fluidity of the membrane. Cholesterol esters and certain carbohydrates are also found in some membranes.

The structure of biological membranes determines their function and characteristics. The most important feature from a toxicological point of view

Introduction to Toxicology

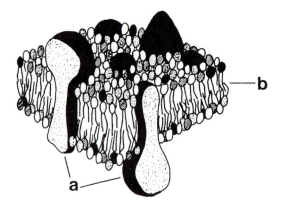

Figure 2.1. The three-dimensional structure of the animal cell membrane. Proteins (a) are interspersed in the phospholipid bilayer (b).

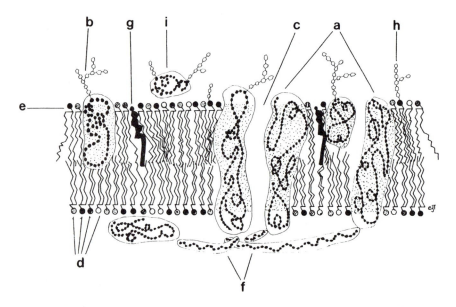

Figure 2.2. The molecular arrangement of the cell membrane. a: integral proteins; b: glycoprotein; c: pore formed from integral protein; d: various phospholipids with saturated fatty acid chains; e: phospholipid with unsaturated fatty acid chains; f: network proteins; g: cholesterol; h: glycolipid; i: peripheral protein. There are four different phospholipids: phosphatidyl serine; phosphatidyl choline; phosphatidyl ethanolamine; sphingomyelin represented as $\bigcirc$; $\odot$; $\oslash$; $\bullet$. The stippled area of the protein represents the hydrophobic portion.

is that they are selectively permeable. Only certain substances are able to pass through them, depending on particular physico-chemical characteristics:

1. size
2. lipid solubility
3. similarity to endogenous molecules
4. polarity/charge

The ways in which foreign substances may pass through biological membranes are as follows:

1. filtration through pores
2. passive diffusion through the membrane phospholipid
3. active transport
4. facilitated diffusion
5. phago/pinocytosis

1. *Filtration*. Small molecules may pass through pores in the membrane formed by proteins. This movement will occur down a concentration gradient and may include substances such as ethanol and urea.

2. *Passive diffusion*. This is probably the most important mechanism of absorption for foreign and toxic compounds. For passive diffusion to occur certain conditions are required:

a. there must be a concentration gradient across the membrane
b. the foreign molecule must be lipid soluble
c. the compound must be non-ionized

These principles are embodied in the pH-partition theory: only non-ionized lipid soluble compounds will be absorbed by passive diffusion down a concentration gradient. Furthermore certain factors affect the rate at which foreign compounds passively diffuse. This rate of diffusion is described by Ficks Law:

$$\text{Rate of diffusion} = KA(C_2 - C_1)$$

where A is the surface area, C_2 is the concentration outside and C_1 the concentration inside the membrane, and K is a constant.

The above relationship applies to a system at constant temperature and for diffusion over unit distance. The concentration gradient is represented by $(C_2 - C_1)$. Passive diffusion is a first order process, that is the rate of diffusion is proportional to the concentration.

Normally biological systems are dynamic and the concentration on the inside of the membrane is continually reducing as the foreign compound is being removed by blood flow and possibly ionization (Figure 2.3). Consequently there is always a concentration gradient towards the inside of the membrane. As well as a concentration gradient, lipid solubility and ionization and, hence, the pH of the particular tissue fluid are also factors in passive diffusion. Lipid soluble compounds are able to pass across biological membranes by dissolution in the phospholipid and movement down the concentration gradient. Ionizable compounds will only do this if they are in

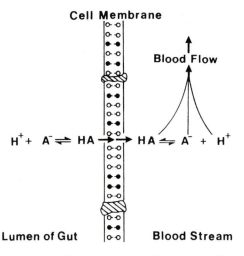

Figure 2.3. Role of blood flow and ionization in the absorption of foreign compounds. Both blood flow and ionization create a gradient across the membrane.

the non-ionized form. The degree of ionization can be calculated from the Henderson Hasselbach equation:

$$pH = pK_a + \frac{Log[A^-]}{[HA]}$$

where pK_a is the dissociation constant for the acid, HA. The ionization of an acid and base are shown in Figure 2.4. The role of ionization will be more fully discussed when the gastrointestinal tract is considered.

3. *Active transport*. Active transport of compounds across membranes has several important features:

    a. a specific membrane carrier is required
    b. metabolic energy is necessary to operate the system
    c. the process may be inhibited by metabolic poisons
    d. the process may be saturated at high substrate concentrations and hence is zero order rather than first order
    e. transport occurs against a concentration gradient
    f. similar substrates may compete for uptake

There are various kinds of active transport systems which involve carrier molecules operating in different ways. These are uniports, symports and antiports. The uniport transports one molecule in a single direction. Symports and antiports transport two molecules in the same or opposite directions respectively.

This type of membrane transport is normally specific for endogenous and nutrient substances but analogues and similar molecules or ions may be

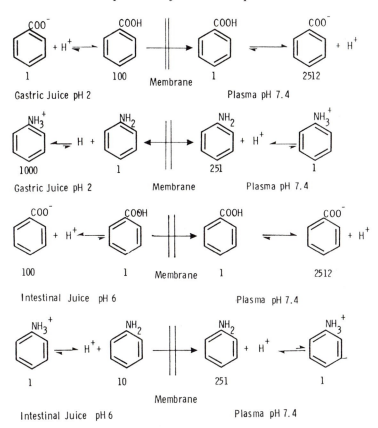

Figure 2.4. Ionization of an acid and base in the stomach and intestine.
From Timbrell, J. A., *Principles of Biochemical Toxicology*, Taylor & Francis, London, 1991.

transported by the system. For example, the drug fluorouracil, an analogue of uracil and lead ions are absorbed from the gut by specific transport systems.

4. *Facilitated diffusion*. This has the following salient features:

   a. a specific membrane carrier is required
   b. a concentration gradient across the membrane is necessary
   c. the process may be saturated by high substrate concentrations

Unlike active transport, no energy expenditure is necessary. This type of transport system also normally applies to endogenous substances and normal nutrients but may apply to foreign compounds which are structurally similar to an endogenous compound. The transport of glucose from the cells of the intestine into the bloodstream involves this type of system.

5. *Phagocytosis and pinocytosis*. These involve the invagination of the membrane to enclose a particle or droplet respectively. This is the mechanism

by which particles of insoluble substances such as uranium dioxide and asbestos are absorbed into the lungs.

Sites of Absorption

There are three major sites for the absorption of foreign compounds: the skin, lungs and gastrointestinal tract. The gastrointestinal tract is the most important in toxicology as most foreign compounds are ingested orally. The lungs are clearly important for all airborne compounds whereas the skin is only rarely a significant site for absorption.

Skin

The skin is constantly exposed to foreign compounds such as gases, solvents, and substances in solution, and so absorption through the skin is potentially an important route. However, although the skin has a large surface area for absorption, its structure is such as to present a barrier to absorption. This is because there is an outer layer of dead cells, a poor blood supply, and the outer cells of the epidermis are packed with keratin (Figure 2.5). Although the dermis below is vascularized, it is several cells thick and this will also inhibit absorption.

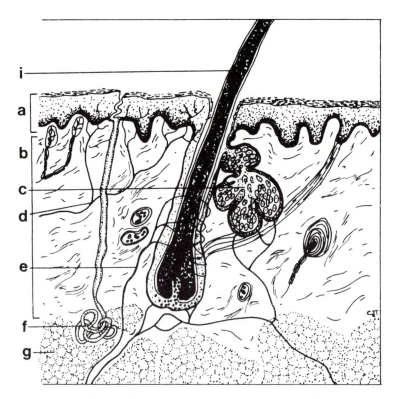

Figure 2.5. The structure of mammalian skin. a: epidermis; b: dermis; c: sebaceous gland; d: capillary; e: nerve fibre; f: sweat gland; g: adipose tissue; i: hair.

Absorption through the skin is mainly limited to lipid soluble compounds such as solvents. Fatalities have occurred, however, following absorption of toxic compounds by this route, such as with the insecticide parathion.

Lungs

Exposure to toxic compounds via the lungs is toxicologically more important than via the skin. The air we breathe may contain many foreign substances. These may be gases (carbon monoxide), vapours from solvents (methylene chloride), aerosols or particulate matter (asbestos) in an industrial or other workplace environment. Also, the air in an urban or home environment may contain noxious gases (sulphur dioxide and nitrogen oxides), particulates (fibre glass and pollen), and possibly solvent vapours and aerosols from home use. The lungs have a very large surface area, around 50–100 m^2 in man, they have an excellent blood supply, and the barrier between the air in the alveolus and the blood stream may be as little as two cell membranes thick (Figure 2.6). Consequently absorption from the lungs is rapid and efficient. Two factors which affect absorption via the lungs are blood flow and breathing rate. For compounds with low solubility in blood the absorption will be mainly dependent on the rate of blood flow. For compounds with high solubility in blood the absorption will be mainly dependent on the breathing rate. The rapid rate

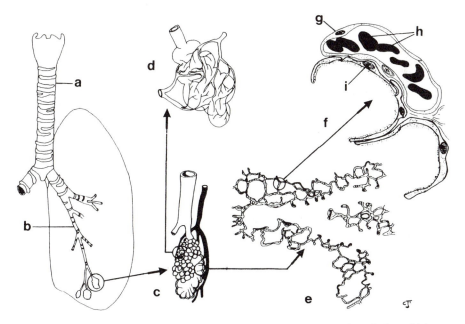

Figure 2.6. The structure of the mammalian respiratory system. a: trachea; b: bronchiole; c: alveolar sac with blood supply; d: arrangement of blood vessels around alveoli; e: arrangement of cells and airspaces in alveoli showing the large surface area available for absorption; f: cellular structure of alveolus showing the close association between the endothelial cell of the capillary, g, with erythrocytes, h, and the epithelial cell of the alveolar sac, i. The luminal side of the epithelial cell is bathed in fluid which also facilitates absorption and gaseous exchange.

of blood flow means that foreign substances are continually removed from the absorption site and, therefore, there is always a concentration gradient. Reaction with plasma proteins and for gases particularly dissolution in the plasma may also be factors.

Small, lipid soluble compounds, such as solvents, will be readily absorbed from the alveolus. For compounds which are absorbed via the lungs it is a very efficient and rapid route of entry to the body. Compounds in solution and particles may be absorbed by pinocytosis and phagocytosis respectively. For example, uranium dioxide particles, which are insoluble, are absorbed via the lungs and cause kidney damage. Lead is also absorbed in the particulate form from the air via the lungs. The size of particle is a major factor in determining where in the respiratory system it is deposited and whether it is absorbed. For example, lead particles of 0.25 μm diameter are absorbed but uranium dioxide particles of more than 3 μm diameter are not.

Gastrointestinal Tract

Numerous foreign substances are taken in via the diet, while many drugs are normally taken by mouth, and various poisonous substances taken either accidentally or intentionally are usually ingested orally. Consequently the gastrointestinal tract is a very important site of absorption for foreign compounds.

The internal environment of the gastrointestinal tract varies throughout its length, particularly with regard to the pH. Substances taken orally first come into contact with the lining of the mouth (buccal cavity), where the pH is normally around 7 in man, but more alkaline in some other species such as the rat. The next region of importance is the stomach where the pH is around 2 in man and certain other mammals. The substance may remain in the stomach for some time particularly if it is taken in with food. In the small intestine where the pH is around 6, there is a good blood supply and a large surface area due to folding of the lining and the presence of villi (Figure 2.7).

Due to the change in pH in the gastrointestinal tract different substances may be absorbed in different areas depending on their physico-chemical characteristics. Lipid soluble, non-ionized compounds will be absorbed along the whole length of the tract, but ionizable substances generally will only be absorbed by passive diffusion if they are non-ionized at the pH of the particular site and are also lipid soluble. The Henderson Hasselbach equation can be used to calculate the extent of ionization of aniline (a weak base) and benzoic acid (a weak acid) at the particular pH prevailing in the stomach and small intestine. It can be seen (Figure 2.4) that weak acids should be absorbed in the stomach and weak bases in the small intestine. However in practice weak acids are also absorbed in the small intestine due to the influence of blood flow and plasma pH. Although they exist mainly in the ionized form in the small intestine (Figure 2.4), the non-ionized form passing into the blood will immediately be removed by:

1. blood flow, and
2. ionization at pH 7.4.

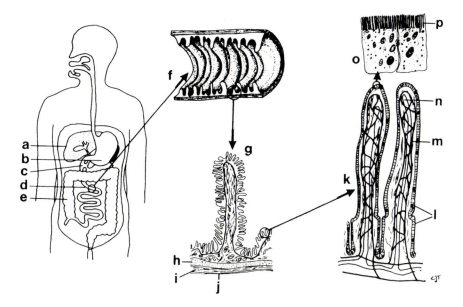

Figure 2.7. The mammalian gastrointestinal tract showing important features of the small intestine, the major site of absorption for orally administered compounds. a: liver; b: stomach; c: duodenum; d: ileum; e: colon; f: longitudinal section of the ileum showing folding which increases surface area; g: detail of fold showing villi with circular and longitudinal muscles, h and i respectively, bounded by the serosal membrane, j; k: detail of villi showing network of capillaries, m, lacteals, n, and epithelial cells, l; o: detail of epithelial cells showing brush border or microvilli, p. The folding, vascularization and microvilli all facilitate absorption of substances from the lumen.

These two factors ensure that weak acids are absorbed to a certain extent in the small intestine if they have not been fully absorbed in the stomach.

Another factor which may affect absorption from the gastrointestinal tract is the presence of food. This may facilitate absorption if the substance in question dissolves in any fat present in the foodstuff but may delay absorption if the compound is only absorbed in the small intestine, as food prolongs gastric emptying time.

When drugs and other foreign compounds are administered the vehicle used to suspend or dissolve the compound may have a major effect on the eventual toxicity by affecting the rate of absorption and distribution.

The site of absorption itself may be important in the eventual toxicity because of the blood supply to that site as discussed in the next section.

The site of absorption and exposure to compounds may also be important in the fate of the compound. For example, the acidic conditions of the stomach may cause the substance to hydrolyze, or poisons such as snake venom may be inactivated. The bacteria in the gastrointestinal tract may metabolize foreign compounds as may enzymes in the gut wall. In the lungs phagocytosis sequesters some inert substances, such as particles of asbestos which can remain in the lung tissue for long periods of time with eventual toxic consequences.

Distribution of Toxic Compounds

After a foreign compound has been absorbed it passes into the bloodstream. The part of the vascular system into which the compound is absorbed will depend on the site of absorption. Absorption through the skin leads to the peripheral blood supply, whereas the major pulmonary circulation will be involved if the compound is airborne and hence absorbed through the lungs. For the majority of compounds oral absorption will be followed by entry of the compound into the portal vein supplying the liver with blood from the gastrointestinal tract.

Once in the bloodstream the compound will then be distributed around the body and be diluted by the blood. Depending on the physico-chemical properties of the compound it may then be distributed into the tissues. As with the absorption of foreign compounds, distribution into particular tissues involves crossing biological membranes and the principles which have already been discussed earlier in the chapter again apply. Only the non-ionized form of compounds will pass out of the bloodstream into tissues by passive diffusion. Specific transport systems may operate for certain compounds, and phagocytosis and pinocytosis may transport large molecules, particles or solutions of large molecules. The concentration of the compound in the plasma and the plasma level profile (Figure 2.8) will reflect the distribution. For example, compounds which are distributed into all tissues, such as lipid soluble solvents like carbon tetrachloride, will tend to have low plasma concentrations, whereas substances which are ionized at the pH of the plasma and which do not readily distribute into tissues, may have much higher plasma concentrations. This can be quantified as the parameter known as apparent volume of distribution, V_D:

$$V_D(L) = \frac{\text{Dose} \quad (mg)}{\text{Plasma concentration (mg L}^{-1})}$$

(There are other means of determining V_D which the interested reader may find in more advanced texts.)

This is the volume of body fluids into which the particular substance is apparently distributed. The determination is analogous to dissolving a known amount (dose) of a substance in an unknown volume of water (body fluids). A knowledge of the concentration of compound in the water (plasma level) allows us to determine the volume of water.

The volume of distribution may sometimes indicate that a foreign compound is localized in a particular tissue or is confined mainly to the plasma. Thus, if a substance distributes mainly into adipose tissue, the plasma concentration will be very low and from the above formula it can be seen that the volume of distribution will be large. The substance is not necessarily evenly distributed in body water however and may reach high concentrations in one particular tissue or organ.

The plasma concentration, or better the area under the plasma concentration versus time curve (AUC) (Figure 2.8) gives a much more meaningful

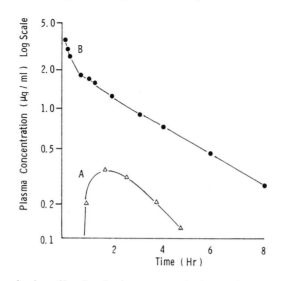

Figure 2.8. Plasma level profile of a foreign compound after oral (A) and intravenous (B) administration. The difference between the profile may indicate first-pass metabolism is occurring. From Timbrell, J. A., *Principles of Biochemical Toxicology*, Taylor & Francis, London, 1991.

indication of the exposure of the animal than the dose as it indicates the concentration to which the tissue or receptor site may be exposed. This is usually the case but there are exceptions such as when a compound is sequestered or concentrated in a tissue. The plasma level also reflects the absorption, distribution, metabolism, and excretion of the compound. It is an essential piece of information for the treatment and management of drug overdoses and during chronic dosing as it may indicate when accumulation is occurring. The plasma level is therefore a very important parameter in toxicology. An indication of the overall exposure of the animal is given by the whole body burden, determined from $V_D \times$ plasma concentration.

Another important value is the half-life of the compound ($t\frac{1}{2}$). This may be the plasma half-life or the whole body half-life and indicates the length of time required for the concentration in the plasma or body to decrease by one half. This may be a very important factor in the toxicity of the compound as a substance with a long half-life can accumulate during chronic exposure. The longer a substance remains in the body of an animal, the more chance for toxic effects to occur. The half-life is determined by both the metabolism and elimination and as both of these processes may be saturable, dose dependent changes in the half-life will indicate saturation of either or both processes.

It will be clear from Figure 2.8 that the AUC after oral dosing is much less than that after intravenous dosing. This may be because the drug or other compound is metabolized during the absorption process either in the gastrointestinal tract or in the liver. This is known as 'first-pass metabolism' and means that less of the parent compound reaches the circulation after oral dosing.

Another indicator of the ability of the body to eliminate the compound is the total body clearance which is calculated as shown:

$$\frac{\text{dose}}{\text{AUC}}$$

(The units are ml min^{-1} if the dose is in mg and the plasma concentration is plotted as mg ml^{-1} against minutes.)

Another aspect of the distribution phase which may have important toxicological implications is the interaction of foreign compounds with proteins in plasma and various macromolecules in other tissues. Many foreign compounds bind to plasma proteins non-covalently and in doing so their distribution is altered. Distribution from the blood into the tissues is reduced by binding to such proteins as the foreign compound is now attached to a large molecule which limits its passage across membranes unless a specific transport system exists. Binding can also limit excretion as will be discussed later. Foreign compounds in plasma often exist in equilibrium between the bound and unbound form and the extent of binding and the tightness of that binding varies between different compounds. Binding may involve ionic forces, hydrogen bonding, hydrophobic bonding and Van der Waals forces. Foreign compounds bind most commonly to albumin but some, such as DDT, which are lipophilic may associate extensively with plasma lipoproteins.

Distribution of foreign compounds to those tissues which may be the site of action is a particularly important aspect of their toxicology. For example, barbiturates act on the central nervous system and so must enter the brain in order to have a pharmacological, and if exaggerated, toxic, effect. The entry of substances into the brain is less readily attainable than passage into other tissues because of the so-called blood-brain barrier. This is due to the nature of the capillaries serving the brain. These are surrounded by cells which do not allow the ready passage of substances into the central nervous system. Lipid soluble compounds such as some of the barbiturates will enter the brain by passive diffusion. However, some barbiturates, such as phenobarbitone, are weak acids and so ionize. In the treatment of barbiturate poisoning this ionization is utilized by increasing the plasma pH with infusions of sodium bicarbonate. This increases the ionization of the barbiturate in the plasma, changes the equilibrium and so causes more unionized drug to diffuse out of the tissues, including the brain, into the plasma. Another compound which is known to be toxic due to its effect on the central nervous system is methyl mercury, a lipophilic mercury derivative which is able to cross the blood-brain barrier.

Lipophilic foreign compounds localize particularly in body fat, sometimes to the extent that the plasma level is hardly detectable and the V_D is very large. For example, polybrominated biphenyls, substances once used extensively in industry, are very persistent and highly fat soluble. This localization in body fat resulting in very long whole body half-lives may have important toxicological consequences. The drug thiopental, a barbiturate anaesthetic which is very lipid soluble, has an extremely rapid onset of action due to its ability to enter the brain very quickly.

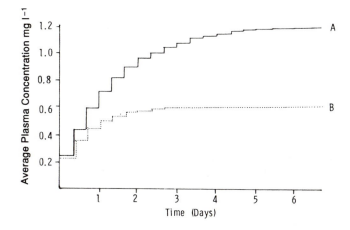

Figure 2.9. Accumulation of two compounds after multiple dosing. Compound A has a half-life of 24 hours, compound B of 12 hours. Dosing interval is 8 hours.
From Timbrell, J.A., *Principles of Biochemical Toxicology*, Taylor & Francis, London, 1991.

Some toxic foreign compounds are chronically ingested or there is continuous exposure to them over shorter periods and this may alter their disposition. If the dosing interval is shorter than the half-life the compound will accumulate in the animal (Figure 2.9). The blood and tissue level may increase disproportionately and dramatically under certain circumstances, such as where excretion or metabolism is saturated. Otherwise the plateau level reached in the plasma is proportional to the plasma half-life, so that compounds with long half-lives could accumulate to significant levels on repeated dosing or exposure despite the low level of each dose or exposure (Figure 2.9).

Excretion of Toxic Compounds

The elimination of toxic substances from the body is clearly an important determinant of their biological effect; rapid elimination will reduce the likelihood of toxicity occurring and reduce the duration of the biological effect. In the case of a toxic effect, removal of the compound may help to reduce the extent of damage.

The elimination of foreign compounds is reflected in either the plasma half-life or the whole body half-life. However, the plasma half-life also reflects metabolism and distribution as well as excretion. The whole body half-life is the time required for half of the compound to be eliminated from the body and consequently reflects the excretion of the compound.

The most important route of excretion for most compounds is through the kidneys into the urine. Other routes are secretion into the bile, excretion into the expired air from the lungs for volatile and gaseous compounds and secretion into the gastrointestinal tract, milk, sweat and other fluids.

Urinary excretion

Excretion into the urine from the bloodstream applies to relatively small, water-soluble molecules; large molecules such as proteins do not pass out through the intact glomerulus and lipid soluble molecules such as bilirubin are reabsorbed from the kidney tubules.

The kidneys receive approximately 25 per cent of the cardiac output of blood and so they are exposed to and filter out a significant proportion of foreign compounds. Excretion into the urine involves one of three mechanisms: filtration from the blood through the pores in the glomerulus; diffusion from the bloodstream into the tubules; and active transport into the tubular fluid.

The structure of the kidney facilitates the elimination of compounds from the bloodstream (Figure 2.10). The basic unit of the kidney, the nephron, allows most small molecules to pass out of the blood in the glomerulus into the tubular ultrafiltrate aided by large pores in the capillaries and the pressure of the blood. Lipid-soluble molecules will passively diffuse out of the blood provided there is a concentration gradient. However, if such compounds are not ionized at the pH of the tubular fluid, they may be reabsorbed from the

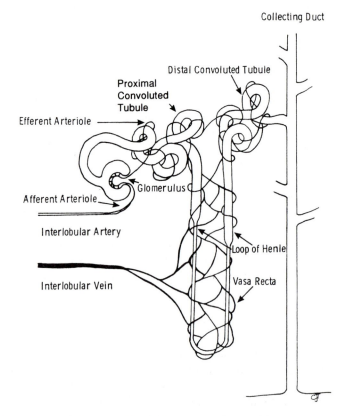

Figure 2.10. Structure of the mammalian kidney.
From Timbrell, J. A., *Principles of Biochemical Toxicology*, Taylor & Francis, London, 1991.

tubule by passive diffusion back into the blood as it flows through the vessels surrounding the tubule because there will be a concentration gradient in the direction tubule → blood. Water-soluble molecules which are ionized at the pH of the tubular fluid will not be reabsorbed by passive diffusion and will pass out into the urine.

Certain molecules, such as p-aminohippuric acid, a metabolite of p-aminobenzoic acid are actively transported from the bloodstream into the tubules by a specific anion transport system.

Passive diffusion of compounds into the tubules is proportional to the concentration in the bloodstream, so the greater the amount in the blood the greater will be the rate of elimination. However, when excretion is mediated via active transport or facilitated diffusion, which involves the use of specific carriers, the rate of elimination is constant and the carrier molecules may become saturated by large amounts of compound. This may have important toxicological consequences. As the dose of a compound is increased, the plasma level will increase. If excretion is via passive diffusion, the rate of excretion will increase as this is proportional to the plasma concentration. If excretion is via active transport, however, increasing the dose may lead to saturation of renal elimination and a toxic level of compound in the plasma and tissues may be reached. This is the case with ethanol where continuous intake leads to ever increasing plasma levels accompanied by the well-known effects on the central nervous system.

Another factor which may affect excretion is binding to plasma proteins. This may reduce excretion via passive diffusion especially if binding is tight and extensive as only the free portion will be able to passively diffuse into the tubule. Protein binding does not affect active transport however and a compound such as p-aminohippuric acid which is 90 per cent bound to plasma proteins is cleared in the first pass of blood through the kidney.

One of the factors which affects excretion is the urinary pH. If the metabolite excreted into the urine is ionizable it may become ionized when it enters the tubular fluid. For example, an acidic drug such as phenobarbital is ionized at alkaline urinary pH and a basic drug such as amphetamine is ionized at an acidic urinary pH. This factor is utilized in the treatment of poisoning by barbiturates. The pH of urine may be affected by diet; high protein diet for instance causes urine to become more acid. The rate of urine flow from the kidney into the bladder is also a factor in the excretion of foreign compounds; high fluid intake, and therefore production of copious urine, will tend to facilitate excretion.

Biliary Excretion

Excretion into the bile is an important route for certain foreign compounds, especially large polar substances. Indeed, it may indeed be the predominant route of elimination. Bile is secreted in the liver by the hepatocytes into the canaliculi and it flows into the bile duct and eventually into the intestine (Figure 2.11). Consequently compounds which are excreted into the bile are usually eliminated in the faeces. Molecular weight is an important factor in

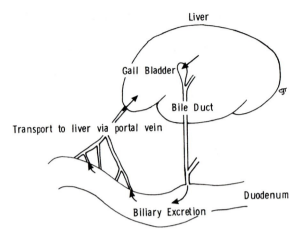

Figure 2.11. Biliary excretion route for foreign compounds.
From Timbrell, J. A., *Principles of Biochemical Toxicology*, Taylor & Francis, London, 1991.

biliary excretion as can be seen from Table 2.1 and so for polar compounds with a molecular weight of 300 or so, such as glutathione conjugates, biliary excretion can be a major route of excretion. Excretion into the bile is an active process and there are three specific transport systems, one for neutral compounds, one for anions and one for cations.

As with renal excretion via active transport, biliary excretion may be saturated and this may lead to an increasing concentration of compound in the liver. For example, the drug furosemide was found to cause hepatic damage in mice due to saturation of the biliary excretion route which caused an increase in its concentration in the liver.

Another consequence of biliary excretion is that the compound comes into contact with the gut microflora. The bacteria may metabolize the compound and convert it into a more lipid-soluble substance which can be reabsorbed from the intestine into the portal venous blood supply and so return to the liver. This may lead to a cycling of the compound known as enterohepatic recirculation which may increase the toxicity (Figure 2.11). If the compound is taken orally, and therefore is transported directly to the liver and is extensively excreted into the bile, it may be that none of the parent compound ever

Table 2.1. Effect of molecular weight on the route of excretion of biphenyls by the rat.

Compound	Molecular weight	% Total excretion Urine	Faeces
Biphenyl	154	80	20
4-Monochlorobiphenyl	188	50	50
4,4'-Dichlorobiphenyl	223	34	66
2,4,5,2',5'-Pentachlorobiphenyl	326	11	89
2,3,6,2',3',6'-Hexachlorobiphenyl	361	1	99

Source: H. B. Matthews (1980), *Introduction to Biochemical Toxicology*, Hodgson and Guthrie (Eds) (New York: Elsevier-North Holland)

reaches the systemic circulation. Alternatively, the gut microflora may metabolize the compound to a more toxic metabolite which could be reabsorbed and cause a systemic toxic effect. Compounds taken orally may also come directly into contact with the gut bacteria. For example, the naturally occurring glycoside cycasin is hydrolyzed to the potent carcinogen methylazoxymethanol by the gut bacteria when it is ingested orally.

Biliary excretion, therefore, may:

1. increase the half-life of the compound;
2. lead to the production of toxic metabolites in the gastrointestinal tract;
3. increase hepatic exposure via the enterohepatic recirculation;
4. be saturated and lead to hepatic damage.

The importance of biliary excretion in the toxicity of compounds can be seen from Table 2.2 which shows that ligation of the bile duct increases the toxicity of certain chemicals many times.

Excretion via the Lungs

The lungs are an important route of excretion for volatile compounds and gaseous metabolites of foreign compounds. For example, about 50–60 per cent of a dose of the aromatic hydrocarbon benzene is eliminated in the expired air. Excretion is by passive diffusion from the blood into the alveolus assisted by the concentration gradient. This is a very efficient route of excretion for lipid-soluble compounds as the capillary and alveolar membranes are thin and in very close proximity to allow for the normal gaseous exchange involved in breathing. There will be a continuous concentration gradient between the blood and air in the alveolus because of the rapid removal of the gas or vapour from the lungs and the rapid blood flow to the lungs. This may be a very important factor in the treatment of poisoning by such gases as the highly toxic carbon monoxide. Compounds may also be metabolized to volatile metabolites such as carbon dioxide for example.

Table 2.2. Effect of bile duct ligation (BDL) on the toxicity of certain compounds.

Compound	LD_{50}; mg/kg		
	Sham operation	BDL	Sham:BDL ratio
Amitryptiline	100	100	1
Diethylstilboestrol	100	0.75	130
Digoxin	11	2.6	4.2
Indocyanine Green	700	130	5.4
Pentobarbital	110	130	0.8

Source: C. D. Klaassen (1974), *Toxicology and Applied Pharmacology*, **24**, 37.

Other Routes of Excretion

Excretion into breast milk can be a very important route for certain types of compounds especially lipid-soluble compounds. Clearly new born animals will be specifically at risk from toxic compounds excreted into milk. For example nursing mothers exposed to DDT secrete it into their milk and the infant may receive a greater dose, on a weight basis, than the mother. Foreign compounds may be secreted into other body fluids such as sweat, tears or semen and certain compounds may be secreted into the stomach or saliva.

Metabolism of Foreign Compounds

As we have seen, foreign compounds absorbed into a biological system by passive diffusion are generally lipid soluble and consequently not ideally suited for excretion. For example, very lipophilic substances such as DDT (Figure 7.1) and the polychlorinated biphenyls are very poorly excreted and hence remain in the animal's body for many years.

After a foreign compound has been absorbed into a biological system it may undergo metabolism (also known as biotransformation). The metabolic fate of the compound can have an important bearing on its toxic potential, disposition in the body and its excretion. The products of metabolism are usually more water soluble than the original compound. Indeed, in animals biotransformation seems directed at increasing water solubility and hence excretion. Facilitating the excretion of a compound means that its biological half-life is reduced and hence its potential toxicity is kept to a minimum. Metabolism may also directly affect the biological activity of a foreign compound. For example, the drug succinylcholine causes muscle relaxation, but its action only lasts a few minutes because metabolism cleaves the molecule to yield inactive products (Figure 2.12). However, in some cases metabolism increases the toxicity of a compound as we shall discuss later in this book. There are numerous examples of this but a well-known one is ethylene glycol which is metabolized to oxalic acid, partly responsible for the toxicity (Figure 2.13).

Metabolism, therefore, is an extremely important phase of disposition as it may have a major effect on the biological activity of that compound, generally by increasing polarity and so water solubility and thereby increasing excretion. For example, the analgesic drug paracetamol (discussed in Chapter 4) has a renal clearance value of 12 ml min^{-1}, whereas one of its major metabolites, the sulphate conjugate, is cleared at the rate of 170 ml min^{-1}.

Therefore, in summary, metabolism leads to:

1. transformation of the molecule into a more polar metabolite;
2. possible increase in molecular weight and size;
3. facilitation of excretion and so elimination from the organism.

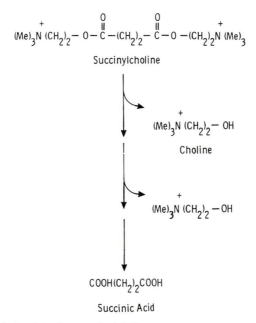

Figure 2.12. Hydrolysis of the drug succinylcholine.
From Timbrell, J. A., *Principles of Biochemical Toxicology*, Taylor & Francis, London, 1991.

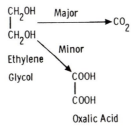

Figure 2.13. Metabolism of ethylene glycol.
From Timbrell, J. A., *Principles of Biochemical Toxicology*, Taylor & Francis, London, 1991.

The consequences of these changes are:

a. the half-life of the compound is decreased;
b. the exposure time is shortened;
c. the possibility of accumulation is reduced;
d. a probable change in biological activity;
e. a change in the duration of the biological activity.

Sometimes metabolism may decrease water solubility and so reduce excretion. For example, acetylation decreases the solubility of sulphonamides in urine and so leads to crystallization in the kidney tubules causing necrosis of the tissue.

Metabolism can be simply divided into two phases: phase 1 and phase 2. Phase 1 is the alteration of the original foreign molecule so as to add on a functional group which can then be conjugated in phase 2. This can best be understood by examining the example in Figure 2.14. The foreign molecule is benzene, a highly lipophilic molecule which is not readily excreted from the animal except in the expired air as it is volatile. Phase 1 metabolism converts benzene into a variety of metabolites, but the major one is phenol. The insertion of a hydroxyl group allows a phase 2 conjugation reaction to take place with the polar sulphate group being added. Phenyl sulphate, the final metabolite is very water soluble and is readily excreted in the urine.

Most biotransformations can be divided into phase 1 and phase 2 reactions, although some foreign molecules already possess functional groups suitable for phase 2 reactions, such as phenol for example. The products of phase 2 biotransformations may be further metabolized in what is sometimes termed phase 3 reactions.

Metabolism is usually catalyzed by enzymes and these are usually, but not always, found most abundantly in the liver in animals. The reason for this location is that most foreign compounds enter the body via the gastrointestinal tract and the portal blood supply goes directly to the liver (Figure 2.7). However, it is important to remember that (1) the enzymes involved with the metabolism of foreign compounds may be found in many other tissues as well as the liver; (2) the enzymes may be localized in one particular cell type in an organ; and (3) the enzymes are not always specific for foreign compounds and may have a major role in normal endogenous metabolism.

The enzymes involved in biotransformation also have a particular subcellular localization: many are found in the endoplasmic reticulum. Some are located in the cytosol and a few are found in other organelles such as the mitochondrion. The various types of metabolic reactions are shown in Table 2.3. For more information on the metabolism of foreign compounds the reader should consult the more detailed texts indicated in the bibliography.

Phase 1 Reactions

Oxidation reactions

The majority of these reactions are catalyzed by one enzyme system, the cytochrome P450 mono-oxygenase system which is located in the smooth endoplasmic reticulum of the cell, isolated as the so-called microsomal fraction obtained by cell fractionation. The liver has the highest concentration of this enzyme although it can be found in most, if not all tissues. The

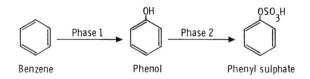

Figure 2.14. Metabolism of benzene.
From Timbrell, J. A., *Principles of Biochemical Toxicology*, Taylor & Francis, London, 1991.

Table 2.3.   The major biotransformation reactions.

Phase 1	Phase 2
Oxidation	Sulphation
Reduction	Glucuronidation
Hydrolysis	Glutatione conjugation
Hydration	Acetylation
Dehalogenation	Amino acid conjugation

reactions catalyzed also require NADPH, molecular oxygen and magnesium, and the overall reaction is shown below:

$$SH + O_2 + NADPH + H^+ \rightarrow SOH + H_2O + NADP^+$$

where S is the substrate.

The sequence of metabolic reactions is shown in Figure 2.15 and involves four distinct steps:

1. addition of substrate to the enzyme;
2. donation of an electron;

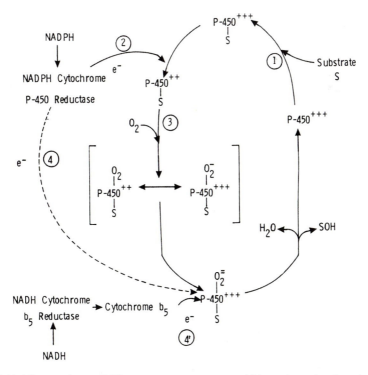

Figure 2.15. The cytochrome P450 mono-oxygenase system which catalyzes the phase 1 metabolism of many foreign compounds.
From Timbrell, J. A., *Principles of Biochemical Toxicology*, Taylor & Francis, London, 1991.

3. addition of oxygen and rearrangement;
4. donation of a second electron and loss of water.

The cytochrome P450 system is actually a collection of isoenzymes all of which possess an iron atom in a porphyrin complex. These catalyze different types of oxidation reactions and under certain circumstances catalyze other types of reaction.

Let us look at the major types of oxidation reaction catalyzed by the cytochrome P450 system.

Aromatic hydroxylation, such as occurs with benzene (Figure 2.14) and aliphatic hydroxylation such as with vinyl chloride (Figure 2.16) involves adding oxygen across a double bond. Hydroxylation of the aliphatic moiety in propylbenzene may occur at one of three positions (Figure 2.17). Alicyclic and heterocyclic rings may also undergo hydroxylation.

Alkyl groups attached to N, O or S atoms may be removed by dealkylation reactions which involve oxidation of the alkyl group and then rearrangement and loss as the respective aldehyde (Figure 2.18). Nitrogen and sulphur atoms in xenobiotics may be oxidized by the microsomal enzymes (Figure 2.19) and sulphur and halogen atoms may be removed oxidatively (Figures 2.20 and 2.21).

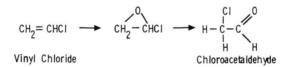

Figure 2.16. Epoxidation of vinyl chloride.
From Timbrell, J. A., *Principles of Biochemical Toxicology*, Taylor & Francis, London, 1991.

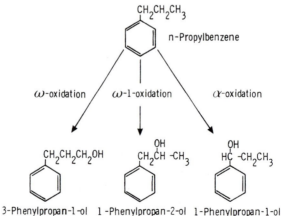

Figure 2.17. Oxidation of n-propylbenzene.
From Timbrell, J. A., *Principles of Biochemical Toxicology*, Taylor & Francis, London, 1991.

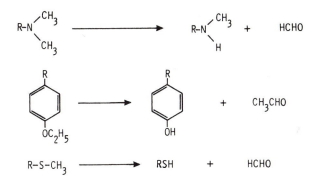

Figure 2.18. Dealkylation reactions.
From Timbrell, J. A., *Principles of Biochemical Toxicology*, Taylor & Francis, London, 1991.

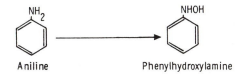

Aniline   Phenylhydroxylamine

Figure 2.19. N-hydroxylation of an aromatic amino group.
From Timbrell, J. A., *Principles of Biochemical Toxicology*, Taylor & Francis, London, 1991.

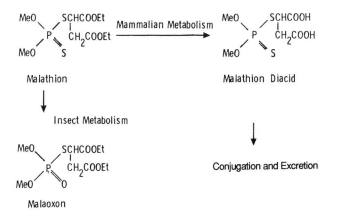

Figure 2.20. Metabolism of the insecticide malathion.
From Timbrell, J. A., *Principles of Biochemical Toxicology*, Taylor & Francis, London, 1991.

Certain oxidation reactions are catalyzed by other enzymes such as alcohol dehydrogenase (Figure 2.22), xanthine oxidase, microsomal amine oxidase, monoamine and diamine oxidases.

Another important group of enzymes which catalyze oxidation reactions for foreign compounds are the peroxidases. For example, the toxic solvent benzene, which causes aplastic anaemia, is believed to be metabolized by peroxidases in the bone marrow. The drug hydralazine is also believed to be metabolized by this enzyme system (see Chapter 4).

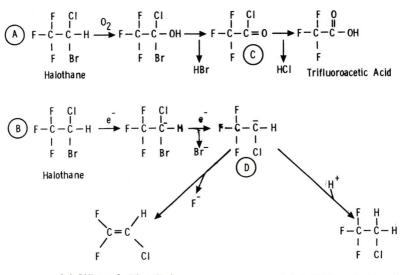

Figure 2.21. Metabolism of the anaesthetic halothane. A is the oxidative pathway, B the reductive pathway. C, trifluoroacetyl chloride is postulated as the intermediate which acylates membrane proteins. D is also a reactive intermediate and may also be involved in reactions with cellular macromolecules and lipid peroxidation.
Adapted from Timbrell, J. A., *Principles of Biochemical Toxicology*, Taylor & Francis, London, 1991.

$$C_2H_5OH \quad \underset{}{\overset{NAD}{\rightleftharpoons}} \quad CH_3CHO \quad \underset{}{\overset{NAD}{\rightleftharpoons}} \quad CH_3COOH$$

Ethanol   Acetaldehyde   Acetic Acid

Figure 2.22. Oxidation of the primary alcohol ethanol.
From Timbrell, J. A., *Principles of Biochemical Toxicology*, Taylor & Francis, London, 1991.

Reduction reactions

These reactions may be catalyzed by either microsomal or cytosolic reductases and by the gut bacteria, which also possess reductases. The most commonly encountered type of reductive reaction is the reduction of nitro and azo groups such as those present in the food colour tartrazine (Figure 2.23). Less common reduction reactions include reduction of aldehyde and keto groups, epoxides and double bonds.

Reductive dehalogenation, catalyzed by the microsomal enzyme system is an important route of metabolism for anaesthetics such as halothane (Figure 2.21) (see Chapter 4).

Reductive dechlorination is involved in the toxicity of carbon tetrachloride.

Hydrolysis

Esters and amides are hydrolyzed by esterases and amidases respectively, and

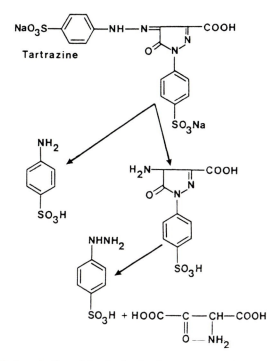

Figure 2.23. Metabolic reduction of the food-colouring agent tartrazine.

there are a number of these enzymes, which are usually found in the cytosol of cells in a variety of tissues. Some are also found in the plasma. Microsomal esterases have also been described. Typical esterase and amidase reactions are shown in Figure 2.24. An example of esterase action which is toxicologically important is that of the hydrolysis of the drug succinyl choline. The very short duration of action of this compound is due to it being very rapidly hydrolyzed in the plasma (see Chapter 4). Amidases have an important role in the toxicity of the drugs isoniazid and phenacetin, where hydrolysis is an important step in the metabolic activation.

Hydration

Epoxides, which can be stable metabolic intermediates, may undergo hydration catalyzed by the enzyme epoxide hydrolase located in the microsomal fraction. This is usually a detoxication reaction as the dihydrodiol products are normally much less chemically reactive than the epoxide.

Phase 2 Reactions

These reactions, also known as conjugation reactions, involve the addition of a polar group to the foreign molecule. This polar group is either conjugated to an existing group or to one added in a phase 1 reaction, such as a hydroxyl

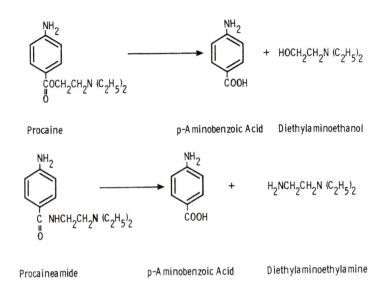

Figure 2.24. Hydrolysis of an ester (the drug procaine) and an amide (the drug procainamide). From Timbrell, J. A., *Principles of Biochemical Toxicology*, Taylor & Francis, London, 1991.

group. The polar group renders the foreign molecule more water soluble and so more readily cleared from the body and less likely to exert a toxic effect. The groups donated in phase 2 reactions are commonly those involved in intermediary metabolism. Conjugation reactions are considered below:

Sulphation

The addition of the sulphate moiety to a hydroxyl group is a major route of conjugation for foreign compounds. It is catalyzed by a cytosolic sulpho-transferase enzyme and utilizes the coenzyme phosphoadenosine phospho-sulphate. The product is an ester which is very polar and water soluble. Both aromatic and aliphatic hydroxyl groups may be conjugated with sulphate as may N-hydroxy groups and amino groups (Figure 2.25).

Glucuronidation

Glucuronic acid is a polar and water soluble carbohydrate molecule which may be added to hydroxyl groups, carboxylic acid groups, amino groups and thiols (Figure 2.26). This process is a major route of phase 2 metabolism and utilizes glucuronosyl transferases, which are microsomal enzymes, with uridine diphosphate glucuronic acid as the cofactor. Other carbohydrates may also be involved in conjugation such as glucose, which is utilized by insects to form glucosides. Ribose and xylose may also be used in conjugation reactions.

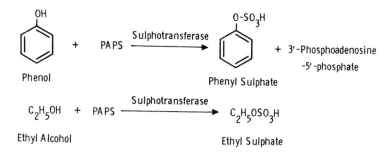

Figure 2.25. Conjugation of a phenol and an aliphatic alcohol with sulphate. PAPS is the sulphate donor, phosphoadenosinephosphosulphate.
From Timbrell, J.A., *Principles of Biochemical Toxicology*, Taylor & Francis, London, 1991.

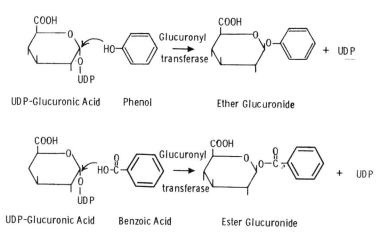

Figure 2.26. Conjugation of a phenol and a carboxylic acid with glucuronic acid.
From Timbrell, J.A., *Principles of Biochemical Toxicology*, Taylor & Francis, London, 1991.

Glutathione conjugation

This is a particularly important route of phase 2 metabolism from the toxicological point of view as it is often involved in the removal of reactive intermediates. Glutathione is a tripeptide found in many mammalian tissues, but especially in the liver. It has a major protective role in the body as it is a scavenger for reactive compounds of various types, combining at the reactive centre in the molecule and so reducing or abolishing the toxicity. Normally, the sulphydryl group of glutathione acts as a nucleophile and either displaces another atom or attacks an electrophilic site (Figure 2.27). Consequently glutathione may react either chemically or in enzyme-catalyzed reactions with a variety of compounds which are either reactive or are electrophilic metabolites produced in phase I reactions. The reactions may be catalyzed by one of a group of glutathione transferases located in the soluble fraction of the cell. They have been detected also in the microsomal fraction. The substrates include aromatic, heterocyclic, alicyclic and aliphatic epoxides, aromatic halogen and nitro compounds and unsaturated aliphatic compounds. The

Introduction to Toxicology

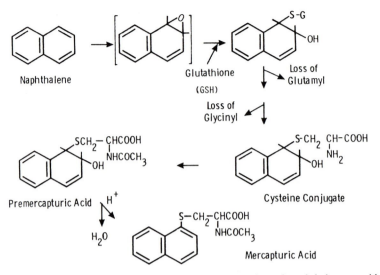

Figure 2.27. Metabolism of napthalene showing the conjugation of naphthalene epoxide with glutathione and the subsequent formation of a N-acetylcysteine conjugate (mercapturic acid). From Timbrell, J.A., *Principles of Biochemical Toxicology*, Taylor & Francis, London, 1991.

conjugate which results may be either excreted into the bile unchanged or metabolized further, via so-called phase 3 reactions, to yield an N-acetylcysteine conjugate or mercapturic acid (Figure 2.27).

Acetylation

This metabolic reaction is unusual in that the product may be less water soluble than the parent compound. Substrates for acetylation are aromatic amino compounds, sulphonamides, hydrazines and hydrazides (Figure 2.28).

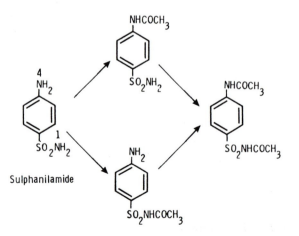

Figure 2.28. The acetylation of the amino and sulphonamido groups of the drug sulphanilamide. From Timbrell, J.A., *Principles of Biochemical Toxicology*, Taylor & Francis, London, 1991.

The enzymes involved are acetyltransferases and are found in the cytosol of cells in the liver, gastric mucosa and white blood cells. The enzymes utilize acetyl Coenzyme A as cofactor. There are two isoenzymes in the rabbit which differ markedly in activity and the same is probably true in humans. In both species the possession of a particular isoenzyme is genetically determined and gives rise to two distinct phenotypes known as 'rapid' and 'slow' acetylators. This has an important role in the toxicity of certain drugs such as hydralazine (see Chapter 4), isoniazid and procainamide, and these examples illustrate the importance of genetic factors in toxicology.

Amino acid conjugation

Foreign organic acids may undergo conjugation with amino acids (as well as with glucuronic acid, see above). The particular amino acid utilized depends on the species concerned and, indeed, species within a similar evolutionary group tend to utilize the same amino acid. Glycine is the most common amino acid used. The carboxylic acid group first reacts with Coenzyme A and then with the particular amino acid. The acylase enzyme catalyzing the reaction is found in the mitochondria.

Methylation

Hydroxyl, amino and thiol groups in molecules may be methylated by one of a series of methyltransferases. This occurs particularly with endogenous compounds but xenobiotics may also be substrates. As with acetylation this reaction tends to decrease rather than increase water solubility.

An important toxicological example is the methylation of heavy metals such as mercury. This may be carried out by micro-organisms in the environment (see Chapter 8). The importance is that this changes the physico-chemical characteristics of mercury from a water-soluble inorganic ion, to a lipid-soluble organic compound. There is also a corresponding change in the toxicity of mercury with mercuric ion being toxic to the kidney in contrast to organomercury which is toxic to the nervous system.

There are other reactions that a foreign molecule may undergo but the interested reader should consult one of the texts or reviews given in the bibliography. One important point to remember, however, is that although a molecule is foreign to a living organism, it may still be a substrate for an enzyme involved in normal metabolic pathways, provided its chemical structure is appropriate, and so this widens the scope of potential metabolic reactions. Foreign compounds can be metabolized by a number of different enzymes simultaneously in the same animal and so there may be many different metabolic routes and metabolites. The balance between these routes can often determine the toxicity of the compound.

Toxication Versus Detoxication

The metabolism of foreign compounds has been termed detoxication because

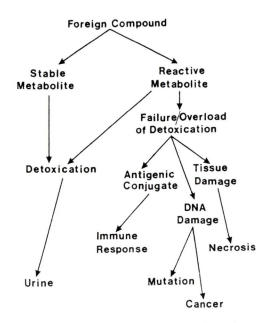

Figure 2.29. An illustration of the ways in which the metabolism of a compound may have a variety of consequences for the organism.

in general it converts these compounds into more water-soluble, readily excreted substances and decreases the toxicity. However, in some cases the reverse occurs and a metabolite is produced which is more toxic than the parent compound. A prime example of this is the drug paracetamol (acetaminophen) which is discussed in more detail in Chapter 4. However, in this case there are several pathways of metabolism that compete. Consequently, factors that alter the balance between these pathways will alter the eventual toxicity. This balance between toxication and detoxication pathways (Figure 2.29) is very important in toxicology and underlies some of the factors that affect toxicity. These will be discussed later in this chapter.

Factors Affecting Toxic Responses

As already indicated, metabolism is a major factor in determining the toxicity of a compound. Factors that affect the disposition will consequently affect toxicity. There are many such factors, which may be either chemical or biological. Chemical factors include the physico-chemical characteristics (pK_a, lipophilicity, size, shape) and chirality (various types of isomers). Biological factors are more numerous and include species, genetics, diet, age, sex, pathological state. Many of these factors affect metabolism and so may influence the toxicity of the compound. For example, different isomers may be metabolized differently and hence show different biological activity. In humans, genetic differences may affect metabolism and consequently toxicity. Different species will have different metabolic capabilities and, therefore, may be more or less susceptible to the toxic effects of some compounds. Dietary constituents may influence metabolic pathways or rate of metabolism and, therefore, whether or not a compound is toxic. However, many of these factors will be discussed and highlighted in examples in later chapters and so will not be discussed in detail here.

Species

Species often vary widely in their responses to toxic compounds and this may be extremely important in relation to veterinary medicine, human medicine and environmental toxicology. For example, drugs are tested in animals for eventual use in man. If the response in the human animal is very different from that in rats or mice problems may arise when the drug undergoes clinical trials.

Similarly, veterinary products may be used on a variety of species and if there are big differences in toxicity this may lead to fatalities or pathological damage in farm animals or pets. In the environment very large numbers of widely different species may all be exposed to a pesticide and may react very differently. Indeed this difference in sensitivity is exploited in pesticides. Insecticides, such as organophosphorus compounds and DDT (see Chapter 7), are much more toxic to insects than to humans and other mammals; in some cases this is due to metabolic differences. For example, the insecticide malathion is metabolized by hydrolysis in mammals but is oxidized in the insect to malaoxon which then binds to and inhibits the enzyme cholinesterase (Figures 2.20 and 7.4; see also Chapter 7).

There are very many species differences in metabolism and it is beyond the scope of this book to discuss them in detail. The interested reader is recommended to consult the bibliography at the end of this chapter.

Strain of Animal

Just as different species may vary in their response to toxic compounds and in the way they metabolize them, different inbred strains of the same animal may also show variation. For example, different strains of mice vary widely in their ability to metabolize barbiturates and consequently the magnitude of the pharmacological effect varies between the strains (Table 2.4).

Sex

Males and females can also differ in their responses due to metabolic and hormonal differences. Males in some species metabolize compounds more rapidly than females, although this difference is not found in all species. As well as metabolic differences there are examples of sex differences in routes of excretion which underlie differences in susceptibility. For example, dinitrotoluene-induced hepatic tumours occur predominantly in males due to the differences in the route of excretion. Biliary excretion of a glucuronide conjugate is favoured in males while urinary excretion predominates in females.

Table 2.4. Strain differences in the duration of action of hexobarbital in mice.

Strain	Sleeping time
A/NL	48 ± 4
BALB/cAnN	41 ± 2
C57L/HeN	33 ± 3
C3HfB/HeN	22 ± 3
SWR/HeN	18 ± 4
Swiss (non-inbred)	43 ± 15

Source: G. E. Jay (1955), *Proceedings of the Society of Experimental Biology and Medicine*, **90**, 378

The glucuronide conjugate is broken down in the intestine by gut bacteria and the products are reabsorbed, causing the hepatic tumours. The difference in susceptibility to chloroform-induced kidney damage between male and female mice is an example of a sex difference which has a metabolic basis and hormonal basis. The male mice are more susceptible but this difference can be removed by castration and restored by androgens. It may be that testosterone is influencing the microsomal enzyme-mediated metabolism of chloroform to give greater metabolism in males.

Genetic Factors and Human Variability in Response

Genetic variation is particularly important in the human population which is genetically mixed. There are now many examples of toxic drug reactions which occur in individuals due to a genetic defect or genetic difference in metabolism. The best known example in man is that of the acetylator phenotype where the acetylation reaction (see page 46) shows genetic variations which are due to mutations giving rise to mutant alleles. This results in rapid and slow acetylators where the latter have less functional acetyltransferase enzyme. This is an important factor in a number of adverse drug reactions including the hydralazine-induced lupus syndrome discussed in Chapter 3, procainamide-induced lupus syndrome, isoniazid-induced liver damage and isoniazid-induced peripheral neuropathy.

Another important genetic factor in metabolism is that shown in the hydroxylation of debrisoquine, the details of which are discussed in Chapter 4. This variation in oxidation has now been shown for a number of other drugs such as phenytoin, sparteine and phenformin. In some cases, toxic reactions are associated with the 'poor metabolizer' status (see Chapter 4).

Toxic responses to foreign chemicals may show large variation between human subjects and some of this variation can be ascribed to the factors mentioned. As well as genetically determined metabolic differences, there may be genetic differences in a receptor or in an immunological parameter giving rise to variation in toxicological and pharmacological responses to drugs and other foreign compounds. Several examples will be discussed later in this book. In some cases, however, rare idiosyncratic reactions of unknown origin may occur and in other cases a combination of factors may be necessary for a toxic reaction to occur (see Chapter 4; hydralazine). Unfortunately, much of the variability seen in humans is not encountered in inbred experimental animals and consequently rare but severe and life-threatening toxic reactions may not be encountered in toxicity studies in animals and may only become known after very large numbers of humans have been exposed to the particular chemical.

Environmental Factors

Another factor which affects the human population is the environment, in particular the other chemical substances to which people are exposed. Thus, chemicals in the diet, air or water may all influence the toxic response to another chemical. Unlike experimental animals, humans may be under medication with several drugs when exposure to an industrial chemical occurs for instance. These drugs can influence the way in which the body reacts to the chemical. The intake of one drug may affect the response to another. For example, overdoses of paracetamol are more likely to cause serious liver damage if the victim is also exposed to large amounts of alcohol or barbiturate, both of which induce drug metabolizing enzymes and thereby increase the *in vivo* activity.

Compounds which inhibit metabolic pathways by blocking particular enzymes may also be factors in toxic responses. For example, workers exposed to the solvent dimethylformamide seem more likely to suffer alcohol-induced flushes than those not exposed, possibly due to the inhibition of alcohol metabolism. The diet contains many substances which may influence the enzymes of drug metabolism such as the microsomal enzyme inducer β-naphthoflavone found in certain vegetables. Cigarette smoking and alcohol intake also are known to affect drug metabolism and pharmacological and toxicological responses.

Pathological State

The influence of disease states on metabolism and toxicity has not been well explored. Diseases of the liver will clearly affect metabolism but different liver diseases can influence metabolism differently. Disease states such as influenza are also known to affect drug metabolizing enzymes, possibly via the production of interferon.

Questions

1. Describe the processes involved in the absorption of chemicals from various named sites of exposure in a mammalian system. Indicate what factors may affect these processes of absorption.

2. Write notes on three of the following:

   (a) volume of distribution;
   (b) first pass effect;
   (c) binding of chemicals to plasma proteins;
   (d) Ficks Law of diffusion.

3. Discuss why a knowledge of the plasma level of a foreign compound is important for a toxicologist. What factors affect the plasma level and what information may be gained from it?

4. Using examples of substrates to illustrate your answers write short notes on three of the following:

   (a) cytochrome P450;
   (b) acetylation;
   (c) glutathione conjugation;
   (d) reduction;
   (e) alcohol dehydrogenase.

5. The compounds shown are hypothetical drugs. Indicate diagrammatically ways in which you think they might be metabolized by mammals. Name the enzyme(s) which catalyze the biotransformations you describe.

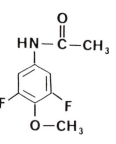
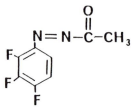
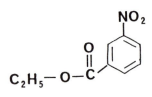

6. Describe the routes and mechanisms involved in the excretion of drugs from the mammalian body. What factors may affect excretion and how might they be toxicologically important?

7. Discuss the role of the physico-chemical properties of chemicals in their disposition.

Bibliography

Ballantyne, B., Marrs, T. and Turner, P. (Eds) (1993) various chapters in Part 1, vol. 1, *General and Applied Toxicology*, Basingstoke: Macmillan.

Bruin, A. DE (1976) *Biochemical Toxicology of Environmental Agents*, Amsterdam: Elsevier.

Caldwell, J. and Jakoby, W. B. (Eds) (1983) *Biological Basis of Detoxication*, New York: Academic Press.

Cassarett and Doull's Toxicology, Amdur, M. O., Doull, J. and Klaassen, C. (Eds) (1991) 4th edition, New York: Pergamon Press.

Clark, B. and Smith, D. A. (1986) *An Introduction to Pharmacokinetics*, 2nd edition, Oxford: Blackwell.

Gibson, G. G. and Skett, P. (1993) *Introduction to Drug Metabolism*, 2nd edition, London: Chapman and Hall.

Hathway, D. E. (1984) *Molecular Aspects of Toxicology*, London: The Royal Society of Chemistry.

Hawkins, D. R. (Ed.) (1988–1993) *Biotransformations*, vols. 1–5, London: The Royal Society of Chemistry.

Hodgson, E. and Levi, P. E. (1987) *A Testbook of Modern Toxicology*, New York: Elsevier.

Hodgson, E. and Levi, P. E. (Eds) (1994) *Introduction to Biochemical Toxicology*, Norwalk, Connecticut: Appleton & Lange.

Hodgson, E., Bend, J. and Philpot, R. M. (Eds) (1979– ●) *Reviews in Biochemical Toxicology*, New York: Elsevier/North Holland.

Jakoby, W. R. (Ed.) (1980) *Enzymic Basis of Detoxification*, New York: Academic Press.

Jakoby, W. R., Bend, J. R. and Caldwell, J. (Eds) (1982) *Metabolic Basis of Detoxification*, New York: Academic Press.

Pratt, W. B. and Taylor, P. (Eds) (1990) *Principles of Drug Action: The Basis of Pharmacology*, 3rd edition, New York: Churchill Livingstone.

Timbrell, J. A. (1991) *Principles of Biochemical Toxicology*, 2nd edition, London: Taylor & Francis.

Williams, R. T. (1959) *Detoxication Mechanisms*, London: Chapman & Hall.

Zbinden, G. (1988) Biopharmaceutical studies, a key to better toxicology, *Xenobiotica*, **18**, suppl. 1, 9.

Chapter 3

Types of Exposure and Response

Types of Exposure

There are two basic exposure conditions for toxic compounds: acute and chronic exposure. Acute exposure applies to a single episode where a particular amount of a substance such as with an overdose of a drug, enters the organism. Chronic exposure applies to repeated exposure to a substance which may then accumulate or cause a cumulative toxic effect.

Acute toxicity usually applies to a toxic event which occurs soon after acute or limited exposure; chronic toxicity may apply to an event which occurs many weeks, months or years after exposure to either repeated doses or possibly after an acute exposure to a particular toxic substance.

Route of Exposure

Routes of exposure have already been discussed in Chapter 2 and so only brief mention will be made here. Exposure via the gastrointestinal tract is the most important route for most drugs, food additives and contaminants, natural products, and other potentially toxic substances. Inhalation is particularly important in an industrial environment both inside and outside the factory and pesticides may also be taken in this way during spraying. Absorption via the skin is also important in an industrial and agricultural setting.

The site and route of absorption is important from two points of view:

1. the route may influence the eventual systemic toxicity as already indicated in Chapter 2;
2. the site may be important if there is local toxicity at the point of absorption.

For example, substances which are irritant may cause inflammation at the site of absorption and this may depend on the conditions at this site. Particles such as asbestos will cause damage to the cells of the lung by being taken up into them, but will not particularly damage the skin. The skin will tend to be more resistant because of the outer layer of keratinized cells and its poor absorptive properties.

Drugs may also gain access to the body by routes other than those mentioned, in particular intravenous and intramuscular injection are employed in human medicine while intraperitoneal and subcutaneous administration are commonly used in experimental animals. Intravenous and intraperitoneal injection lead to rapid distribution to most parts of the body whereas subcutaneous and intramuscular injection usually lead to slow absorption.

Types of Toxic Response

A biological system may respond in many different ways to a toxic compound. As already mentioned in the section on the dose response relationship death of the cell or of the whole organism is only one response and there are many specific causes of this. We will briefly consider the types of response here and examples will be considered in more detail in later chapters.

The major toxic responses observed are as follows: tissue damage and other pathological changes; biochemical lesions; pharmacological responses or physiological changes; reproductive or teratogenic effects; mutagenicity; carcinogenicity; irritation and corrosive effects; allergic reactions. Clearly there is overlap between some of these responses. For example, biochemical effects can lead to tissue damage or some other pathological lesion. (See paracetamol, Chapter 4 and snake venoms, Chapter 9.)

Direct tissue damage is usually the result of cellular destruction. This may have a biochemical or immunological basis but many pathological lesions are of unknown mechanism, particularly as regards the intermediate stages between the interaction of the toxin or its metabolite with cellular constituents and the start of the final degenerative changes leading to cell death. Highly reactive compounds may react with cell membranes and cause instant cell death by damaging the cell membrane sufficiently to allow rapid loss of contents and influx of external ions and substances. Some toxic compounds interfere directly with vital cellular functions such as respiration which usually leads to rapid cell death. Not all toxic compounds act in this way, however, and some cause cell death to occur more slowly. (See lead, Chapter 8.)

Biochemical lesions may lead to the development of a pathological change such as cell degeneration but they may also simply cause death of the whole organism by interfering with some vital function such as respiration. For example, cyanide causes death of cells by interfering with the electron transport chain in the mitochondria such that oxygen cannot be utilized leading to the death of cells in vital organs so that the whole organism dies. Some biochemical effects are reversible, such as the binding of carbon monoxide to haemoglobin which may be insufficient to cause death of either cells or the whole organism and generally will not result in a pathological lesion (see carbon monoxide and also ethylene glycol, Chapter 10).

Pharmacological and physiological responses are those where a particular bodily function is affected. For example, some compounds cause a change in blood pressure by affecting β-adrenoceptors or by causing vascular dilatation or constriction. These clearly are toxic reactions if extreme and directly life threatening or when they occur in workers occupationally exposed to the drug for example. Alternatively, a drop in blood pressure may be sufficient to initiate another response such as ischaemic tissue damage due to insufficient blood flow. (See debrisoquine and succinyl choline, Chapter 4 and tetrodotoxin and botulinum toxin, Chapter 9.)

Allergic reactions are those that occur when the immune system of the body is stimulated to react in a particular way. This may be the result of a toxic molecule being sufficiently large to be regarded as foreign by the immune system and so act as an antigen. More commonly the foreign compound (or hapten as it is called) interacts with an endogenous macromolecule (usually a protein) and the product, often a conjugate of the hapten and protein, is antigenic (Figure 3.1). An immunological reaction takes one of several forms including stimulation of a physiological response such as bronchoconstriction or cellular destruction by complement. An immunologically mediated reaction may underly a rare, idiosyncratic, response after exposure to a toxic compound,

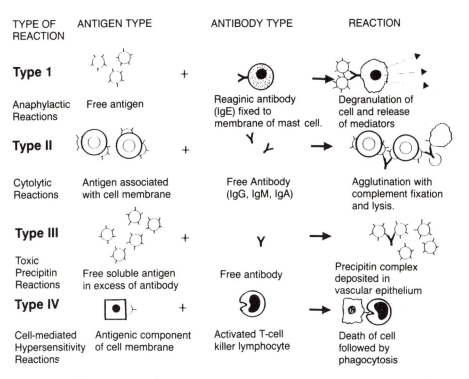

TYPE OF REACTION	ANTIGEN TYPE	ANTIBODY TYPE	REACTION
Type 1 Anaphylactic Reactions	Free antigen	Reaginic antibody (IgE) fixed to membrane of mast cell.	Degranulation of cell and release of mediators
Type II Cytolytic Reactions	Antigen associated with cell membrane	Free Antibody (IgG, IgM, IgA)	Agglutination with complement fixation and lysis.
Type III Toxic Precipitin Reactions	Free soluble antigen in excess of antibody	Free antibody	Precipitin complex deposited in vascular epithelium
Type IV Cell-mediated Hypersensitivity Reactions	Antigenic component of cell membrane	Activated T-cell killer lymphocyte	Death of cell followed by phagocytosis

Figure 3.1. Mechanisms for the stimulation of an immune response. The antigen is usually a foreign macromolecule such as a protein or an altered cell membrane as in Type IV reactions. Most foreign compounds are of low molecular weight and are not directly antigenic. They may act as haptens and so cause immune reactions by reacting with and thereby altering endogenous proteins or cell membrane components.
Adapted from Bowman, W. C. and Rand, M. J., *Textbook of Pharmacology*, 2nd edition, Blackwells Scientific Publishers, Oxford.

such as halothane (see Chapter 4) or it may be cause a more common adverse effect to a drug such as hydralazine (see Chapter 4; also see vinyl chloride Chapter 5). It should be noted that there may be other causes of rare, idiosyncratic, reactions to foreign compounds such as a reduced ability to metabolize a compound (see debrisoquine, Chapter 4).

There are four different types of allergic or hypersensitivity reactions but these will not be discussed in detail in this book. Type I reactions (anaphylaxis) may be elicited by chemicals such as toluene di-isocyanate, an industrial chemical. Sensitization occurs after the initial exposure and then subsequent exposures cause the anaphylactic reaction resulting in bronchoconstriction and asthma. Penicillin may also cause this type of reaction. Type IV reactions underly contact dermatitis which is a major industrial problem associated with exposure to nickel and cadmium.

Most chemical induced adverse skin reactions are probably associated with irritation, and skin disease is the most common injury to industrial chemicals. After a single insult to the epidermis, the primary response is a local inflammatory reaction. Acute inflammation is the immediate response to irritant chemicals and it is characterized by dilation of blood vessels, increased blood flow, accumulation of fluid in the tissues and invasion of white blood cells. These changes give rise to redness, heat, pain and swelling.

Corrosive chemicals such as sodium hydroxide, cause destruction of tissue (see Chapter 10).

Teratogenicity is a very specific type of toxic response whereby the development of the embryo or foetus is affected. This may lead to a functional and/or structural abnormality of the foetus and of the resulting animal. In many cases this is the result of a perturbation in the development of the organism rather than direct damage to the embryo or foetus as the latter usually results in death and abortion. Teratogens are often relatively non-toxic to the mother but interfere in some specific way with the development of a particular stage of the embryo. The timing of the exposure or dosing with a teratogen relative to the stages of pregnancy is therefore crucial (Figure 3.2; see thalidomide, Chapter 4).

Mutagenicity is a toxic effect which specifically damages the genetic material in the cell. The DNA or chromosome is damaged in such a way that an error is transferred to the daughter cell or next generation. Damage to the chromosomes is known as clastogenicity. There are many ways in which a compound may cause a mutation and consequently many different types of foreign compound have been found to be mutagenic. Thus, chemically reactive compounds, such as alkylating agents, may react directly with the DNA in the cell nucleus, or a compound, such as bromouracil, may be incorporated into the DNA during cell replication. This may then lead to mistakes occurring in the new DNA. Some compounds such as the naturally occurring vinca alkaloids interfere with the processes of mitosis or meiosis so that incorrect cell division results. In mammals mutations in the germ cells can lead to birth defects. Mutations in somatic cells are also believed to underlie the development of cancer in most instances (see below).

The majority of human cancers are probably caused by chemical carcinogens

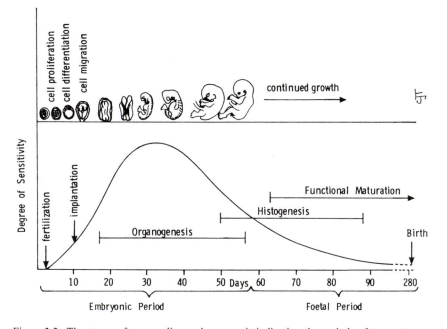

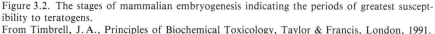

Figure 3.2. The stages of mammalian embryogenesis indicating the periods of greatest susceptibility to teratogens.
From Timbrell, J. A., Principles of Biochemical Toxicology, Taylor & Francis, London, 1991.

and although this is still a contentious issue, there are now many examples of chemicals which will reproducibly cause cancer in experimental animals. Carcinogenicity is a specific toxic effect which leads to the uncontrolled proliferation of tissue. It comes in many different forms, differing in malignancy and type of tissue affected. Cancer induction is now believed to be a multi-stage process which in simple terms requires initiation followed by promotion. Thus, toxic compounds may be carcinogenic by interfering with the genetic control of cellular processes via a mutation, such as the chemically reactive alkylating agents, vinyl chloride and aflatoxins (see Chapter 5 and Chapter 9 respectively). This initiating event is then followed by promotion either by the same compound or some other substance to which the animal is exposed. For example, tumours of mouse skin may be caused by application of a polycyclic hydrocarbon such as benzpyrene (initiator) followed by a phorbol ester (promoter). However, not all carcinogens are mutagens, for example ethionine and asbestos (see Chapter 5). Therefore, mechanisms which do not involve a mutagenic event (epigenetic mechanisms) must be invoked to explain the causation of cancer by such compounds. Also, not all mutagens are carcinogens, although there is a sufficiently good correlation between mutagenicity and carcinogenicity for mutagenicity tests to be regarded as predictive of at least potential carcinogenicity (see Chapter 11). Mutagenicity tests are also of use for prediction of germ cell defects and hence of damage which is heritable.

Detection of Toxic Responses

Some of the toxic effects described may be detected by gross pathological examination in the post mortem or histopathological examination after toxicity studies have been carried out. Some may also be detected using clinical chemical analysis of body fluids, as will be discussed briefly in Chapter 11. The detection of other toxic effects such as mutagenicity may require special techniques.

Thus, toxic responses may be detected in a variety of ways and there is increasing interest in this field of biomarkers. The term biomarkers covers both indicators of effect and exposure. Exposure markers will include the metabolites of the compound in question and conjugates between metabolites and macromolecules such as proteins. There is a wide range of markers of effect such as enzymes released into the blood by damaged tissue, induction of enzyme synthesis or stress proteins and changed synthesis or increased release of various intermediary metabolites. There are also indirect markers of effect such as changes in the immune system or changes in populations resulting from effects on the reproductive cycle of the organism.

Question

1. There are several different types of toxic response which may be caused by chemicals. Describe them and indicate how they can be detected.

Bibliography

Ballantyne, B., Marrs, T. and Turner, P. (Eds) (1993) various chapters in Parts 4 and 5., vols. 1 and 2, *General and Applied Toxicology*, Basingstoke: Macmillan.

Cassarett and Doull's Toxicology, Amdur, M. O., Doull, J. and Klaassen, C. (Eds) (1991) chapters 5–17, 4th edition, New York: Pergamon Press.

Glaister, J. R. (1986) *Principles of Toxicological Pathology*, London: Taylor & Francis.

Greally, J. F. and Silvano, V. (Eds) (1983) *Allergy and Hypersensitivity to Chemicals*. WHO, Copenhagen; CEC, Luxembourg.

Hodgson, E. and Levi, P. E. (Eds) (1994) *Introduction to Biochemical Toxicology*, 2nd edition, Appleton and Lange: Norwalk, Connecticut.

Lu, F. C. (1991) *Basic Toxicology*, 2nd edition, Washington DC: Hemisphere.

Pratt, W. B. and Taylor, P. (Eds) (1990) *Principles of Drug Action: The Basis of Pharmacology*, 3rd edition, New York: Churchill Livingston.

Timbrell, J. A., Draper, R. and Waterfield, C. J. (1994) Biomarkers in toxicology: new uses for some old molecules. *Toxicology and Ecotoxicology. News*, 1, 4–14.

Timbrell, J. A. (1991) *Principles of Biochemical Toxicology*, 2nd edition, London: Taylor & Francis.

Williams, G. M. and Weisburger, J. H. (1986) Chemical carginogens, in *Toxicology: The Basic Science of Poisons*, edited by C. D. Klaassen, M. O. Amdur and J. Doull, New York: Macmillan.

Chapter 4

Drugs as Toxic Substances

'There are no safe drugs, only safe ways of using them.'

'Doctors put drugs of which they know little, into our bodies of which they know less, to cure diseases of which they know nothing at all'.

Voltaire

Introduction

Most human beings and indeed many other animals are exposed to drugs sooner or later in their lives. However, drugs are substances designed to have biological activity and although the layman expects them to be perfectly safe it is not surprising that toxic effects do sometimes occur especially when drugs are wrongly used. However, drugs have made and will continue to make a major contribution to human health and we must accept a measure of risk attached to these benefits.

The tragedy which first made the public and probably also the medical profession fully aware of this unpleasant fact was that caused by the drug thalidomide. This event, perhaps more than any other, proved to be a major watershed for awareness of drug toxicity and the need for better legislation and testing of pharmaceuticals. Consequently, we will consider this as one of our examples which will also serve to illustrate the problem of teratogenesis.

There are several different types of drug toxicity: adverse effects or side effects occurring during proper therapeutic usage; acute toxicity due to overdosage; idiosyncratic reactions which occur during proper therapeutic usage but rarely; interactions with other drugs or other substances being taken concurrently which lead to toxic effects; and habitual abuse of drugs leading to chronic toxicity. Drug overdoses come within the bounds of clinical toxicology as does accidental ingestion of hazardous substances whereas abuse of drugs including their use for murder is the domain of the forensic toxicologist.

The basic mechanisms underlying these types of toxicity may also be summarized:

1. direct and predictable toxic effects due to altered or inhibited metabolism and occurring after overdoses;

2. toxic effects occurring after repeated therapeutic doses with a metabolic, pharmacological or maybe immunological basis;
3. direct but unpredictable toxic effects occurring after single therapeutic doses and due to idiosyncratic metabolism or a pharmacodynamic response;
4. toxic effects due to another drug or substance interfering with the disposition or pharmacological response of the drug in question.

Examples of some of these types of drug toxicity will be considered in this chapter.

Paracetamol

Overdosage with drugs is now one of the commonest means of committing suicide and one of the drugs most commonly involved in the UK is paracetamol with at least 200 deaths a year being due to overdoses of this drug. As well as intentional, suicidal overdoses, accidental poisoning has also occurred and recently been highlighted. This occurred as a result of patients and doctors being unaware that some proprietary preparations contain paracetamol. Thus, repeated self medication with paracetamol tablets possibly along with cold cures which may also contain the drug has lead to fatal overdosage in at least one case (see *Pharmaceutical Journal*, Bibliography). Paracetamol is a minor analgesic which is very safe provided only the normal therapeutic dose of one or two tablets (500 mg) is taken. However, after overdoses, where fifteen or twenty tablets may be taken, fatal liver damage can result. Fortunately an understanding of the mechanism underlying paracetamol toxicity has led to a method of antidotal treatment which is now able to prevent the fatal outcome in many cases.

Paracetamol is metabolized mainly by conjugation with sulphate and glucuronic acid. Only a minor proportion is metabolized by oxidation which is catalyzed by the microsomal mono-oxygenases (Figure 4.1). This produces a metabolite which is toxic but is normally detoxified by reaction with glutathione (see Chapter 2). However, research in experimental animals has shown that after an overdose several changes take place in this metabolic scheme. The pathways of conjugation are saturated and cofactors, especially sulphate, are depleted. As a result more paracetamol is metabolized by the oxidative pathway giving rise to the toxic metabolite. Sufficient of this metabolite is produced in the liver to deplete all the glutathione available. Therefore, the toxic metabolite reacts with liver proteins instead of the glutathione and this causes direct tissue damage leading to hepatic necrosis.

Another factor of importance in relation to the susceptibility to toxicity is individual variation in metabolism, possibly as a result of the intake of other drugs. For example, excessive alcohol intake prior to paracetamol overdose may increase the liver damage as a result of induction of the particular isoenzyme of cytochrome P450 involved in the metabolic activation of paracetamol. The elucidation of this mechanism suggested a means of treatment

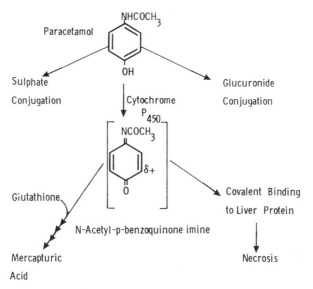

Figure 4.1. The metabolism of the analgesic drug paracetamol.
From Timbrell, J. A., *Principles of Biochemical Toxicology*, Taylor & Francis, London, 1991.

with an antidote to either regenerate glutathione or replace it with an alternative. The currently accepted treatment uses N-acetylcysteine given either orally or intravenously. Provided this is given within 10–12 hours of the overdose fatal liver damage is usually avoided.

A number of other drugs are taken in overdose for purposes of suicide and these cause various toxic effects. Such drugs include aspirin, tranquillizers, barbiturates and opiates but antidotes are not available for most of these. Supportive measures, decreasing absorption, increasing elimination or altering the distribution of the drug are the major types of treatment.

Hydralazine

The second example is of a drug toxicity which follows normal therapeutic dosage leading to adverse effects in a significant number of patients. This example is of particular interest because it illustrates the importance of the combination of several factors in the development of and susceptibility to an adverse drug effect.

The drug in question is the antihypertensive drug hydralazine. This drug causes a syndrome known as lupus erythematosus which has some similarities with rheumatoid arthritis. When the drug was first introduced in the 1950s, relatively high doses were used and the incidence of the adverse effect was high, occurring in over 10 per cent of patients. The use of the drug declined. However, use of lower doses in combination therapy reduced the incidence of the adverse effect although a recent report estimates that the true incidence is still unacceptably high with an overall value of 6.7 per cent. Recent studies have revealed that there are several factors which predispose patients to this particular adverse effect.

The factors so far defined are:

1. dose
2. acetylator phenotype
3. HLA type
4. sex
5. duration of therapy

We will examine each in turn.

Dose

This has already been mentioned. The incidence of the adverse effect seemed to be more common when doses of around 800 mg daily were used compared with doses of less than 200 mg daily, which are more commonly used now. One recent study showed more clearly that the incidence was dose related; as no cases were reported at doses of 50 mg daily, there was a 5.4 per cent incidence after 100 mg daily and a 10.4 per cent incidence with 200 mg daily.

Acetylator phenotype

Hydralazine is metabolized by the acetylation route which is a phase 2 metabolic transformation for foreign compounds which have an amine, sulphonamide or hydrazine group (see Chapter 2). This acetylation reaction is under genetic control in man and human populations can be divided into individuals of the rapid or slow acetylator phenotype. With hydralazine the adverse effect occurs almost exclusively in slow acetylators. As hydralazine undergoes acetylation it is probable that these differences in metabolism of the drug are responsible for the development of the syndrome. It may be that there is more of the parent drug available in slow acetylators which may initiate an immunological reaction. Alternatively, another pathway of metabolism may become more important in the slow acetylators (Figure 4.2). There is some evidence for this with the oxidative pathway, catalyzed by the mono-oxygenases being the most likely route. However there is now evidence that other enzymes, notably peroxidases such as those found in leucocytes are also able to activate hydralazine to yield the same metabolites (phthalazine and phthalazinone). However, which, if any, metabolite is responsible for the adverse effect is currently unknown.

HLA type

It was found that the patients who suffered the syndrome were more likely to have the HLA type (tissue type) DR4 than those not affected. That is, the incidence of HLA DR4 is 60 per cent in those patients with hydralazine induced lupus compared to an incidence of DR4 in the normal population of

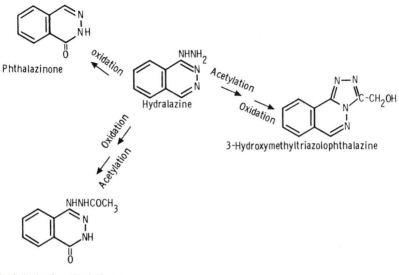

Figure 4.2. The metabolism of the antihypertensive drug hydralazine.
From Timbrell, J. A., *Principles of Biochemical Toxicology*, Taylor & Francis, London, 1991.

27 per cent. The role, if any of the HLA type in the development of the syndrome is currently unknown; it may simply be a marker which has an association with a gene involved in the predisposition for the disease.

Sex

The adverse effect occurs more commonly in women than in men with a sex ratio of about 2:1 overall. However, one recent report quoted an incidence of 19.4 per cent in women taking 200 mg daily compared with an incidence in men of 4.9 per cent when measured three years after starting therapy. Currently there is no explanation for this sex difference as there is no evidence for any difference in acetylator phenotype or HLA type distribution between males and females nor for any difference in metabolism between males and females.

Duration of treatment

The final factor is the duration of treatment with the drug; it seems to require an average of 18 months' treatment for the development of the syndrome.

In view of these factors, the hydralazine-induced lupus syndrome is a particularly interesting example of an adverse drug reaction. The recognition of the predisposing factors allows an estimation of the likely incidence: the HLA type DR4 occurs in around 27 per cent of the population; females account for approximately 50 per cent; slow acetylators are approximately 50 per cent of the British population. Given a sufficiently high dose and duration of treatment these factors give an expected incidence of at least 7 per cent of the normal population. Although true incidence figures are hard to come by, the overall incidence in males and females as recently published is about 10 per cent. Alternatively, it can be regarded thus: a female, slow acetylator with the HLA type DR4 is very likely to suffer the adverse effect if a sufficient dose of the drug is given. This means that the adverse effect could be easily avoided if the prospective patients were screened for HLA type and acetylator phenotype.

The mechanism of hydralazine toxicity is currently unknown although it clearly has features characteristic of an allergic type of reaction. In fact, the adverse effect is usually manifested as a Type III immune reaction (see above, Figure 3.1).

Halothane

An example of an adverse drug effect which is a very rare, idiosyncratic, reaction is afforded by the widely used anaesthetic halothane. This may cause serious liver damage in between 1 in 10 000 and 1 in 100 000 patients. A mild liver dysfunction is more commonly seen but this probably involves a different mechanism.

The predisposing factors so far recognized in halothane hepatotoxicity are:

1. multiple exposures, which seem to sensitize the patient to future exposures;
2. sex, females being more commonly affected than males in the ratio 1.8:1;
3. obesity, 68 per cent of patients in one study were obese;
4. allergy, a previous history of allergy was found in one third of patients.

There is now good evidence that halothane causes hepatic damage via an immunological mechanism. The antibodies bind to the altered liver cell membrane and then killer lymphocytes attach to the antibodies. In response to this the killer lymphocytes lyze and destroy the liver cells of the patient, so causing hepatitis (Figure 4.3). The reactive metabolite involved in the immunological reaction is believed to be trifluoroacetylchloride which acylates proteins. This takes place in the vicinity of the endoplasmic reticulum and consequently enzymes such as cytochrome P450 are believed to be acylated and become antigenic. Such antigens have been identified in liver.

The more common mild liver dysfunction is thought to be due to a direct toxic action of one of the halothane metabolites on the liver. The exact nature of the toxic metabolite is currently unclear although there is some evidence that the metabolite involved in the direct toxicity could either be a product of reductive or oxidative metabolism (Figure 2.21).

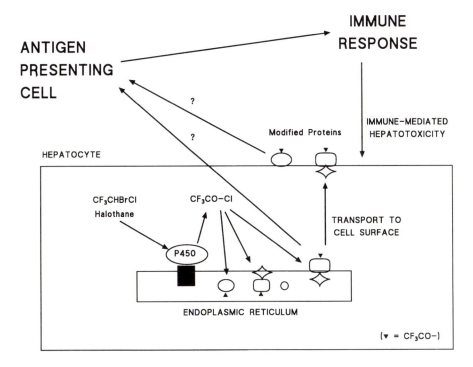

Figure 4.3. The hypothetical mechanism of hepatotoxicity of the anaesthetic drug halothane. Halothane is metabolized by cytochrome P450 (P450) to a reactive metabolite (CF₃COCl) the trifluoroacetyl part of which binds covalently to proteins in the endoplasmic reticulum (▾). The metabolite-protein conjugates are antigenic and elicit immune responses in susceptible patients. Adapted from Kenna, J. G. and Van Pelt, F. N. A. M. (1994) *Anaesth. Pharmacol. Rev.* **2**, 29.

As with hydralazine the knowledge of predisposing factors, in this case the extra risks after multiple exposures, should allow a reduction in the incidence of this adverse drug effect.

The examples used so far have involved a direct toxic effect on tissues mediated either directly or via an immunological mechanism and leading to pathological lesions. The next example illustrates a type of adverse drug reaction in which a pharmacological effect is involved again with a genetic factor.

Debrisoquine

Debrisoquine is a little used antihypertensive drug which was found to show marked inter-individual variation. After the normal recommended therapeutic dose is given this drug may cause an exaggerated pharmacological effect, namely an excessive fall in blood pressure in a few individuals who have a particular genetic predisposition. It has been discovered that about 5–10 per cent of the white population of Europe and North America have this genetic predisposition and are known as poor metabolizers of debrisoquine. This is due to a defect in the mono-oxygenase system which catalyzes the hydroxylation of debrisoquine at the 4 position, the major metabolic reaction (Figure 4.4). Poor metabolizers have almost complete absence of the cytochrome P450 isozyme which catalyzes the hydroxylation of debrisoquine.

As this metabolic reaction is the major route for removal of the drug from the body, such patients have higher plasma levels of the unchanged drug after a normal therapeutic dose than normal subjects. As debrisoquine itself is responsible for the hypotensive effect the result is an excessive fall in blood pressure (Figure 4.5). This is another example of unexpected toxicity occurring in a small proportion of the patients exposed. In this case, however, the metabolic mechanism seems fairly clear.

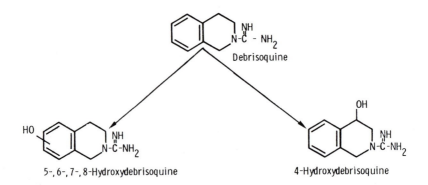

Figure 4.4. The metabolism of the antihypertensive drug debrisoquine.
From Timbrell, J. A., *Principles of Biochemical Toxicology*, Taylor & Francis, London, 1991.

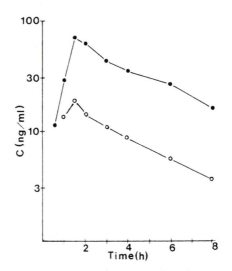

Figure 4.5. The plasma concentration (C) of debrisoquine after a single oral dose (10 mg) in human subjects of the extensive (○) and poor (●) metabolizer phenotypes.
Data from Sloan *et al.* (1983) *British Journal of Clinical Pharmacology*, **15**, 443.

A similar example is the genetically determined toxicity of succinylcholine. This again results from reduced metabolism in certain individuals due to an enzyme variant. Succinylcholine is a muscle relaxant which normally is rapidly removed by metabolic hydrolysis and its duration of action is correspondingly short. In individuals with a defect in the cholinesterase enzyme responsible for the hydrolysis, however, metabolism is slow and consequently relaxation of muscle is excessive and prolonged.

Thalidomide

Thalidomide became notorious as the drug which caused limb deformities in children born to women who had used the drug during pregnancy. The drug is now a well established human teratogen. The thalidomide disaster is particularly important as it was the watershed for drug safety evaluation because it was perhaps the first major example of drug-induced toxicity. Thalidomide is a sedative drug, which was sometimes used for the treatment of morning sickness, and which seemed to be relatively non-toxic. However, it eventually became apparent that its use by pregnant women was associated with a very rare and characteristic limb deformity known as phocomelia in which the arms and legs of the infant were foreshortened. It became clear that these deformities were associated with the use of thalidomide on days 24–29 of pregnancy. The malformations were initially not reproducible in rats or rabbits and had not been detected in the limited toxicity studies carried out by the company manufacturing the drug. The mechanism underlying the effect is still not understood. Thalidomide is an unstable molecule and gives rise to a number of polar metabolites which are derivatives of glutamine and glutamic acid but the ultimate toxic metabolite has not yet been identified. Interestingly one of the isomers of thalidomide (the S-enantiomer) is more embryotoxic than the other. This is an illustration of the importance of chirality as a chemical factor affecting toxicity which has only relatively recently been recognized.

Thalidomide is an exceptionally potent teratogen, but because it has very low maternal toxicity in humans and low toxicity to experimental animals it was allowed to be marketed and used as a drug by pregnant women. It was detected as the cause of the deformities from epidemiological data, when an astute physician associated the exceedingly unusual effects with use of the drug.

There are many other examples of adverse drug reactions which can be found in the literature and the interested reader should consult the references given in the bibliography at the end of this chapter.

Drug Interactions

The problem of interactions between drugs is a major one, particularly with the growth in polypharmacy and multiple drug prescribing. Although the physician and the pharmacist should be aware of such interactions new and unexpected interactions can and do appear. Interactions may be due to any one of a number of mechanisms, such as interference in the metabolism of one drug by another, interference in the disposition of one drug by another or alteration of the pharmacological response to one drug by another.

Many drugs may interfere with the metabolism of another drug either by inducing or inhibiting the enzymes involved (see Chapter 2). The best known example is that of barbiturates, such as phenobarbital, which induce the mono-oxygenase enzymes and so, by altering the rate or route of metabolism of other drugs, may alter their toxicity. Paracetamol overdoses are more severe if such inducing drugs have been taken, because metabolism via the toxic pathway catalyzed by the microsomal mono-oxygenases is enhanced (see above). Enzyme induction may also decrease the pharmacological or toxicological effects of a compound. For example, use of the antitubercular drug rifampicin, which is also a microsomal enzyme inducer, increases the metabolism of contraceptive steroids and so reduces their efficacy, sometimes resulting in unwanted pregnancies. Whether the toxicity of a particular drug will be increased or decreased will depend on the particular drugs involved and the mechanism of the toxic effect.

Interference in the disposition of one drug by another is a common interaction, particularly involving displacement of a drug from a binding site, typically from binding to plasma proteins. A well-known example of this is the displacement of the anticoagulant warfarin from plasma protein binding sites by phenylbutazone, an anti-inflammatory drug. This results in an elevated plasma level of warfarin leading to excessive anticoagulant activity and haemorrhage.

Altered Responsiveness: Glucose-6-phosphate Dehydrogenase Deficiency

Occasionally drug toxicity may occur in some individuals due to an unusual sensitivity, i.e. idiosyncrasy. Perhaps the best known example of this is the acute, drug-induced haemolytic anaemia due to a deficiency in the enzyme glucose-6-phosphate dehydrogenase. This enzyme, which has a major role in intermediary metabolism in the pentose phosphate pathway, is important in maintaining the NADPH concentration in the red blood cell. NADPH is necessary for maintaining the level of reduced glutathione in the red cell, which in turn protects the red cell from oxidizing substances such as the metabolites of certain drugs:

$$GSSG + NADPH + H^+ \rightarrow 2GSH + NADP^+$$

$$\text{Glucose-6-phosphate} + NADP^+ \xrightarrow{G6PD} \text{6-phosphogluconate} + NADPH$$

Patients who have this particular genetic defect suffer acute haemolytic anaemia when they take drugs such as the antimalarial primaquine or are exposed to certain types of foreign compounds such as aniline derivatives.

Fava beans contain a substance which will precipitate haemolytic anaemia in susceptible individuals, hence the term favism.

The deficiency in glucose-6-phosphate dehydrogenase activity is the result of variants in the enzyme rather than complete absence. The enzyme variants are intrinsic to the red blood cell and so red blood cells from victims will be responsive *in vitro*. On challenge with a suitable drug these red blood cells will lyze and it can be shown that the level of glutathione is lower than in non-sufferers and in fact the glutathione level shows a bimodal distribution. It is a genetic defect carried on the X chromosome, so it is sex-linked but the inheritance is not simple. Overall 5–10 per cent of Negro males suffer the deficiency and will suffer acute haemolytic anaemia if challenged with drugs such as primaquine. The highest incidence (53 per cent) is found in male Sephardic Jews from Kurdistan. There are many compounds which will cause haemolytic anaemia in susceptible individuals, some of which require metabolism to reactive metabolites, others not.

Abuse of drugs, alcohol and certain volatile solvents is becoming increasingly common in modern society and consequently so also is toxicity due to this abuse. It is widely known that repeated use of certain drugs leads to habituation and with some drugs to addiction. In some cases the social and related effects of this addiction may be sufficient to indirectly lead to morbidity and death. In other cases actual pathological damage may result as is the case with cocaine which causes liver damage and may also destroy the nasal passages when inhaled. The toxic effects of chronic alcohol abuse on the liver and brain are widely known as are the many hazards of smoking tobacco. Both alcohol and tobacco are addictive drugs and cause far more widespread damage to public health than the more notorious hard drugs such as heroin and cocaine. Drug abuse also causes indirect effects on human health, such as injury following driving under the influence of drugs, child abuse occurring as a result of drug use, and the AIDS virus spreading via intravenous drug users.

Questions

1. Discuss the role of genetic factors in drug toxicity. Use examples to illustrate your answer.
2. 'An understanding of the mechanism underlying the toxicity of paracetamol led to a means of treatment for overdoses.' Explain this statement.

Bibliography

Davies, D. M. (Ed.) (1991) *Textbook of Adverse Drug Reactions*, Oxford: Oxford University Press.

D'Arcy, P. F. (1993) Pharmaceutical Toxicology, in Ballantyne, B., Marrs, T. and Turner, P. (Eds) *General and Applied Toxicology*, Basingstoke, UK: Macmillan.

Dukes, M. N. G. (Ed.) (1977–) *Side Effects of Drugs Annual*, Amsterdam: Excerpta Medica.

Dukes, M. N. G. (Ed.) (1980) *Meylers Side Effects of Drugs*, 9th edition, Amsterdam: Excerpta Medica.

Griffin, J. P. and D'Arcy, P. (1986) *Iatrogenic Diseases*, Oxford: Oxford University Press.

Letter and comment in *Pharmaceutical Journal*, (1992) Paracetamol labelling, Kaye, D. F., page 111; Call for more information on OTC medicines, page 114.

Timbrell, J. A. (1991) *Principles of Biochemical Toxicology*, 2nd edition, London: Taylor & Francis.

Weck, A. L. de and Bundgaard, H. (Eds.) (1983) *Allergic Reactions to Drugs*, Berlin: Springer Verlag.

Chapter 5

Industrial Toxicology

Industrial Chemicals

Industrial diseases have existed ever since man began manufacturing on a large scale, and during the industrial revolution occupational diseases became common. Some were well known to the general public and are still known by their original, colloquial names. These diseases were, and some still are of great importance socially, economically and medically. Many occupations carry with them the risk of a particular disease or group of diseases. Thus, mining has always been a hazardous occupation and miners suffer silicosis, while asbestos workers suffer asbestosis and mesothelioma, and paper and printing workers are prone to diseases of the skin. A man spends on average one-third of his life at work and, therefore, the environment in that workplace can be a major factor in determining his health. Although the working environment has improved immeasurably over the last century, some occupations are still hazardous despite legislation and efforts to improve conditions.

There are now many thousands of chemical substances used in industry ranging from metals and inorganic compounds to complex organic chemicals. The people who work in the industries which use them are therefore at risk of exposure. Fortunately, exposure is often minimized by using chemicals in closed systems so that operators do not come into contact with them, but this is not always the case. In Third World countries, however, some of which are rapidly industrializing, exposure levels are higher and industrial diseases are more common than in the fully developed countries. Consequently exposure to toxic substances in the workplace is still a very real hazard. Furthermore even in the best regulated industrial environment, accidents may happen and can lead to excessive exposure to chemicals.

Means of Exposure

Just as with environmental exposure, exposure in the workplace may occur via any or all of the three major routes: by oral ingestion, by inhalation, and by absorption following skin contact. The most common routes of exposure are, however, via inhalation and skin contact. These routes of exposure apply to gases, vapours, aerosols, volatile solvents and other liquids as well as to dusts and fibres. The skin and lungs may come into contact with substances in all of these states and the substances can either be absorbed or cause local toxic effects.

Toxic Effects

The toxic effects of industrial chemicals may be either chronic or acute. The acute inhalation of solvents in large quantities can cause asphyxiation, unconsciousness or death, for example. Inhalation of large quantities of very irritant substances, such as methyl isocyanate for instance, may cause immediate bronchoconstriction and pulmonary oedema leading to death. Both of these pulmonary effects are locally mediated rather than systemic effects. However, such acute effects are usually accidental and so are probably less common than the chronic industrial diseases. They may cause subsequent chronic toxicity, however.

Inhalation of some chemicals, such as industrial gases, metal fumes or organic solvents, leads to irritation or damage to the respiratory tract which may be acute or chronic. In the long term cancer or debilitating respiratory diseases may result. In the acute phase irritation and allergic responses may occur. Absorption of substances via the lungs is efficient and rapid and may lead to systemic effects such as narcosis from solvents or kidney damage from metal salts such as uranium dioxide.

Exposure of the skin to some substances in the workplace may cause local irritation, whilst others can lead to contact dermatitis or other types of chronic skin disease. Some compounds may be absorbed through the skin and cause toxic effects elsewhere in the body. For example, the insecticide parathion has been known to cause fatal poisoning following skin absorption.

As might be expected the respiratory system and skin are the organs most commonly affected by industrial chemicals. Indeed, the most prevalent occupational disease is dermatitis and this accounts for more working days lost in the UK than all other prescribed (see Glossary) industrial diseases together. Dermatitis may have many causes including exposure to organic and inorganic chemicals. Furthermore, chemical agents may act simply as irritants or they may be sensitizers. In some cases the symptoms may be similar such as the induction of inflammation for example. The number of primary irritants is large and includes many different types of chemical substance such as acids, alkalies, metals and solvents and solid organic and inorganic chemicals. Many of these substances will affect the skin in different ways: solvents will degrease skin, whereas acids and alkalies will denature skin proteins.

Skin sensitizers act via an immunological mechanism to cause contact dermatitis. The chemical may pass through the epidermis and react with proteins such as keratin, to produce an antigen. This 'foreign', antigenic protein then initiates the production of antibodies. Re-exposure to the substance will then initiate an allergic reaction. There are a large number of sensitizers of many different chemical types as shown in Table 5.1. Nickel and its salts are

Table 5.1. Types of skin sensitizers

Type	Chemical class/example
Dye intermediaries	Aniline compounds
Dyes	p-Phenylenediamine
Photographic developers	Hydroquinone
Anti-oxidants	o- and p-toluidine
Insecticides	Organophosporus compounds
Resins	Urethane
Coal tar derivatives	Anthracene
Explosives	Picric acid
Metals	Nickel, Chromium

a well-known cause of contact dermatitis (nickel itch). This may result from occupational exposure and also from exposure to nickel in jewellery.

Sensitization may also be a problem following inhalation exposure where it may lead to a systemic effect such as asthma. Toluene-diisocyanate is a pulmonary sensitizer which is widely used in industry.

Some compounds such as the chlorinated hydrocarbons cause occupational acne, which results from plugging of the pores and increased production of keratin.

Vinyl Chloride

Vinyl chloride or vinyl chloride monomer (VCM) as it is commonly known is the starting point in the manufacture of the ubiquitous plastic polyvinyl chloride (pvc). This plastic was introduced a number of years ago and there have been many workers exposed or potentially exposed to vinyl chloride during the course of their working lives. However, safety standards in factories and working practices have not always been as rigorous as they are today and were perhaps not always observed. In some cases workers were required to enter reaction vessels periodically to clean them, despite the fact that they still contained substantial traces of vinyl chloride. As vinyl chloride is a gas it can be inhaled but is also readily absorbed through the skin. This was sufficient for some of the workers to be overcome by solvent narcosis. The chronic toxic effect of this was not immediately apparent but the most severe lesion, a liver tumour known as haemangiosarcoma, was very rare and was observed only in epidemiological studies of workers in this industry. This tumour was generally confined to workers exposed to extremely high concentrations of vinyl chloride. This type of liver tumour has now also been produced in experimental animals. The hygiene and safety standards applied to working with vinyl chloride are now stricter. However, this occurred with the benefit of hindsight and with more foresight the tragedy might have been avoided.

Chronic exposure to vinyl chloride results in 'vinyl chloride disease' which comprises Raynauds phenomenon (see Glossary), skin changes, changes to the bones of the hands, liver damage and in some cases haemangiosarcoma. The bone changes are due to ischaemic damage following degeneration and occlusion of small blood vessels and capillaries. The liver may become fibrotic. It has been suggested that the vinyl chloride syndrome has an immunological basis, as immune complexes are deposited in vascular epithelium and complement activation is a feature.

The toxic effects of vinyl chloride may result in part from metabolic activation, as it is metabolized by cytochrome P450 to the reactive intermediates, chloroethylene oxide or chloroacetaldehyde, which alkylate DNA and this may thereby lead to cancer (Figure 2.16). The metabolism is saturable and the incidence of liver tumours produced in animals reaches a maximum. The tumour incidence therefore correlates with the amount of vinyl chloride metabolized rather than the dose. The reactive intermediate may also react with other macromolecules and cause the tissue damage seen either directly or via an immunological reaction.

The lessons from this example are that safety standards need to be stringent in factories and that animal studies are important in assessing potential toxicity and highlighting the type of toxic effect that might be expected. This should be known before human exposure occurs. As a consequence of this type of industrial problem legislation is now in force in most major Western countries which deals specifically with industrial chemicals. For example, in the UK all chemicals produced in quantities of greater than 1 tonne have to undergo toxicity testing (see Chapter 11), whilst strict occupational hygiene limits, known variously as Maximum Exposure Limits (MEL; UK) or Threshold Limit Values (TLV; USA) for industrial chemicals are enforced.

Cadmium

Cadmium is a metal which is widely used in industry in alloys, in plating, in batteries and in the pigments used in inks, paints, plastic, rubber and enamel. It is also found naturally and may be present in food although it is poorly absorbed from the gut (5–8 per cent). However, up to 40 per cent of an inhaled dose is absorbed and therefore the presence of cadmium in cigarette smoke is more significant. It is an extremely toxic substance and the major hazard is from inhalation of cadmium metal or cadmium oxide. Cadmium has many toxic effects, primarily causing kidney damage, as a result of chronic exposure, and testicular damage after acute exposure, although this does not seem to be a common feature in humans after occupational exposure to the metal. It is also a carcinogen in animals causing tumours in the testes as well as at the site of exposure.

Kidney damage may be a delayed effect even after single doses, being due to the accumulation of cadmium in the kidney, as a complex with the protein metallothionein. Metallothionein is a low molecular weight protein involved with the transport of metals within the body. Due to its chemical similarity to zinc, cadmium exposure induces the production of this protein and 80–90 per cent of cadmium is bound to it *in vivo*. The cadmium-metallothionein complex is transported to the kidney, filtered through the glomerulus and is reabsorbed by the proximal tubular cells. Within these cells the complex is degraded by proteases to release cadmium which may damage the cells or recombine with more metallothionein.

The testicular damage occurs within a few hours of a single exposure to cadmium and results in necrosis, degeneration and complete loss of spermatozoa. The mechanism involves an effect on the vasculature of the testis. Cadmium reduces blood flow through the testis and ischaemic necrosis results from the lack of oxygen and nutrients reaching the tissue. In this case cadmium is probably acting mainly indirectly by affecting a physiological parameter.

The half-life of cadmium in the body is between 7 and 30 years and it is excreted through the kidneys, particularly after they become damaged.

After acute inhalation exposure lung irritation and damage may occur along with other symptoms such as diarrhoea and malaise while chronic inhalation exposure can result in emphysema occurring before kidney damage is observed. Cadmium can also cause disorders of calcium metabolism and the subsequent loss of calcium from the body leads to osteomalacia and brittle bones. In Japan this became known as Itai-Itai ('Ouch-Ouch!') disease when it occurred in women eating rice contaminated with cadmium.

Aromatic Amines

Aromatic amines are widely used in the rubber and dye industry and cause various toxic effects. β-Naphthylamine, which was formerly used in the rubber industry is one of the few compounds known to be a human carcinogen causing bladder cancer. It was withdrawn from industrial use in 1949. The earliest cases of bladder cancer due to aromatic amines were reported in Germany in 1895 amongst aniline dye workers.

There are a number of different aromatic amines used in industry (Figure 5.1) and some of them are known to be carcinogenic at least in animals.

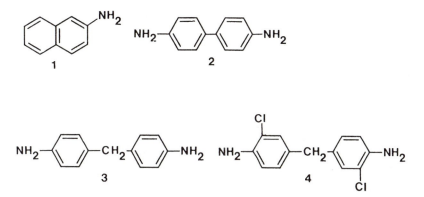

Figure 5.1. The structures of some carcinogenic aromatic amines. 1: 2-naphthylamine; 2: benzidine; 3: 4,4′-diamino-diphenylmethane (DADPM); 4: 3,3′-dichloro-4,4′-diamino-diphenyl-methane, (4,4′-methylene-bis-(2-chloroaniline, MBOCA)).

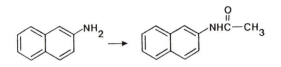

Figure 5.2. The acetylation of 2-naphthylamine.

However, β-naphthylamine has been extensively studied and serves as an example. The mechanism of the bladder cancer is believed to involve metabolism. β-Naphthylamine undergoes hydroxylation at the nitrogen atom followed by conjugation of the resulting hydroxyl group with glucuronic acid (Figure 2.26). When the conjugate is excreted into the urine, however, it breaks down under the acidic urinary conditions to yield a reactive metabolite which can then react with cellular macromolecules such as DNA.

It has recently been proposed that the acetylator phenotype may be a factor in bladder cancer induced by aromatic amines. Acetylation is one route of detoxication for these compounds (Figure 5.2) and consequently slow acetylators would be exposed to more of the aromatic amine than rapid acetylators.

Other aromatic amines used in industry which are carcinogenic in animals are methylene-*bis-o*-chloroaniline (MBOCA), benzidine, *o*-tolidine, 4-aminobiphenyl and diaminodiphenylmethane (DADPM) (Figure 5.1). This latter compound was responsible for an outbreak of jaundice in the UK, which became known as Epping Jaundice. A solution of the chemical was spilt onto the floor of a lorry which subsequently carried sacks of flour. These became contaminated with the substance and people who ate the bread made from this flour became ill with jaundice. DADPM causes bile duct damage and liver tumours in rodents rather than bladder tumours. The target organ for the aromatic amines, however, seems to depend on the species as in rodents' liver tumours generally result whereas in the dog bladder tumours occur more often.

Workers who are occupationally exposed to aromatic amines should undergo cytological examination of urine as well as other screening procedures. Aniline, the simplest aromatic amine, causes methaemoglobinaemia and consequently cyanosis after acute exposure. After chronic exposure anaemia with mild cyanosis may occur.

Asbestos

The industrial diseases associated with exposure to asbestos illustrate that even chemically inert substances can be very toxic. The term asbestos covers a group of fibrous mineral silicates which have differing chemical compositions. It is widely used in industry because of its ability to withstand heat and to provide insulation. Chrysotile (white asbestos) is the form most commonly used and is relatively inert biologically but crocidolite (blue asbestos) and a common contaminant of white asbestos is especially hazardous as it may cause mesothelioma, a rare form of cancer, and also bronchial carcinoma (cancer of the lung).

It has been estimated that deaths due to asbestos will peak at between 2–3000 per year in the UK and 10 000 per year in the US over the 30-year period from 1983. There have been more than 400 known deaths from mesothelioma alone in the UK and this cancer is solely associated with exposure to asbestos. Extensive exposure is normally via inhalation in factories manufacturing asbestos products or during its use as an insulating material, such as in power stations and in warships during the Second World War. More recently, workers have been exposed potentially to asbestos during the demolition of buildings in which it has been used. It is widely used in brake linings. The general population is also exposed to asbestos in food and water. It has been used as a material for filters and, hence, may appear in drinks, and it occurs in drinking water in some areas where mining takes place. However, the toxicological importance of this route of exposure is currently uncertain, but gastrointestinal tumours have been ascribed to asbestos after inhalation exposure.

Exposure to asbestos via inhalation can lead to the following conditions:

1. Asbestosis or interstitial fibrosis of the lung;
2. Benign pleural disease;
3. Bronchial carcinoma;
4. Malignant mesothelioma.

Asbestosis is a dose-related disease and requires heavy exposure for a prolonged period. Particles of asbestos can be detected in the fibrotic areas of the lung and sputum and the air spaces become obliterated with collagen. The asbestos fibres become coated with an iron-containing protein. The disease develops over a variable period of time with breathlessness becoming more severe. Monitoring the lung function of exposed workers in some way, such as by measuring vital capacity, should be carried out as a consistent reduction could indicate the effects of asbestos exposure.

Although asbestos is chemically inert, the fibres are cytotoxic and will haemolyze red blood cells. The length of the fibre seems to be an important factor in the toxicity—fibres which are longer than 10–20 μm will cause fibrosis but shorter ones do not. This is due to the inability of macrophages to phagocytose the long fibres fully and so the macrophage cell membrane is damaged and enzymes leak out. These enzymes and other cellular constituents may be involved in the development of fibrosis. The lung normally can remove hazardous particles but the long asbestos fibres are not adequately removed and as already indicated they are also not effectively removed by macrophages. An immunological mechanism is also involved and asbestos fibres cause a change in the cell surface of the macrophage after ingestion. This is a change in the receptors for C_3 complement and IgG antibodies. The complement pathway is also activated.

In the UK there is legislation to control the use of asbestos and workers must have a medical examination before and at regular intervals during their exposure. Crocidolite is no longer used in the UK, the use of amosite (brown asbestos) is not encouraged, and the general use of asbestos for insulation will probably be banned. The control limit for crocidolite and amosite in the environment is 0.2 fibres per ml and 0.5 fibres per ml for other forms of asbestos.

Bronchial carcinoma may result from prolonged exposure to asbestos and occurs in approximately 50 per cent of those workers who develop asbestosis. As well as the dose and duration of exposure, the type of exposure is also important. The use of asbestos products, such as in textiles, where asbestos of a particular particle size is generated is probably important in the development of the disease.

Mesothelioma is a rare form of cancer which affects the chest lining and is associated only with exposure to asbestos, especially but not exclusively, crocidolite. Crocidolite from the north-west Cape Province in South Africa is more potent than that from the Transvaal. Prolonged exposure to high levels of asbestos is not necessary for the development of mesothelioma and it has developed in people not occupationally exposed to asbestos. Although the latent period is usually long, typically 30 years after exposure, once diagnosed the disease is usually fatal within months rather than years. The tumour may eventually spread to the lung and may eventually encase it.

The mechanisms underlying asbestos-induced cancer are currently unknown but do not seem to involve genotoxic mechanisms. Animal studies as well as human data have shown that asbestos fibres alone will cause cancer of the mesothelium. Unlike other types of chemical carcinogen, asbestos is not metabolized or activated *in vivo* but once present in the tissues it remains there permanently although the fibres do migrate from the airways to the pleural cavity. Consequently, even exposure to high levels for short periods of time may be sufficient to eventually cause mesothelioma.

The size of the fibres appears to be a critical factor, with those 0.3 μm in diameter and 5 μm in length being the most active. The extent of exposure in terms of the concentration of fibres in inhaled air is also important. Other factors have also been identified. There may be a synergistic effect between smoking and asbestos in the induction in pulmonary carcinogenesis.

Legislation

In the UK, the USA and in most other major Western industrialized nations there is legislation which sets limits on the levels of toxic substances in the workplace. This involves setting exposure levels based on the results of human epidemiological data and on the results of animal toxicity studies. It requires monitoring of the occupational environment for compliance. The experimental evidence of toxic effects usually includes, the determination of a dose-response relationship and no-effect levels in experimental animals. Limited studies, such as exposure to solvents for irritant effects, for skin sensitization may, however, be conducted in human volunteers under carefully controlled conditions after ethical considerations have been made.

The maximum level of exposure for a compound is known as the Maximum Exposure Limit (MEL) in the UK or the threshold limit value (TLV) in the

USA. These are calculated on the basis of exposure over a normal working day usually from a knowledge of the toxicity of the compound in experimental animals (NOAEL) with a margin of safety included in the estimate (see Chapters 1 and 11). Such occupational exposure limits are set by the regulatory body, in the case of the UK this is the Health and Safety Executive, and these should not be exceeded. The fact that industrial diseases still occur suggests that some factories do not adhere to these limits or that safety precautions such as the wearing of masks are not taken. Unfortunately with some diseases, such as cancer, the development time is long and therefore diseases may occur many years after the initial, critical exposure when safety standards were not as strict as those today.

This long latency period also means that the detection of industrial diseases is often difficult, as there has to be a sufficient rarity and sufficiently increased frequency of the disease within a particular population for epidemiologists to detect it. In the UK however, new legislation requires all new chemical substances not already covered by existing legislation (drugs and pesticides) to undergo toxicological testing and consequently exposed people can be screened for the likely toxic effects. In addition, it allows hazards to be identified so that control measures, such as suitable labelling, can be effected. Despite this, however, new occupational diseases will undoubtedly continue to appear resulting from exposure many years ago. Also, new and unexpected toxic effects may also occur.

Question

1. Write notes on the toxicity of the following:

   (a) vinyl chloride;
   (b) asbestos;
   (c) aromatic amines.

Bibliography

Anderson, K. E. and Scott, R. M. (1981) *Fundamentals of Industrial Toxicology*, Ann Arbor, Mich.: Ann Arbor Science.
Hamilton, A. and Hardy, H. L. (1983) *Industrial Toxicology*, revised A. J. Finkel, Bristol: J. Wright & Sons.
Hunter, D. (1978) *Diseases of Occupations*, 6th edition. London: Hodder & Stoughton.
Lauwerys, R. R. (1991) Occupational Toxicology, in *Cassarett and Doull's Toxicology*, Amdur, M. O., Doull, J. and Klaassen, C. (Eds), 4th edition, New York: Pergamon Press.
Patty's Industrial Hygiene and Toxicology (1978) vols I–III, 3rd edition, New York: John Wiley.
Stacey, N. (Ed.) (1993) *Occupational Toxicology*, London: Taylor & Francis.
Waldron, H. A. (1985) *Lecture Notes on Occupational Medicine*, 3rd edition, Oxford: Blackwell.

Chapter 6

Food Additives and Contaminants

Introduction

The food we consume daily contains many different substances, some natural, some added intentionally and some present due to contamination. Substances intentionally added to food, 'food additives', are not as recent an innovation as is often supposed; the use of salt as a preservative and spices to disguise poor food has been common for centuries. However, such treatment of food with additives has only reached the current scale relatively recently, with something of the order of 2500 food additives currently in use. The use of food additives on such a wide scale is now beginning to be questioned by some toxicologists especially as the long-term effects of the substances in question often are not known. The general public also now questions the use of some of these additives and in response to this food manufacturers have begun to supply certain foods which are additive-free or contain only 'natural' colouring agents.

Food additives, grouped according to their use with some examples, are shown in Table 6.1. It can be seen that as well as the colouring agents and preservatives there are other types of additive whose function is less obvious. In Europe, permitted food additives are given a number, the E number, which also appears on the packaging of the food.

Food additives have many functions but primarily they allow the consumer to buy food at his convenience and the producer to 'improve' the quality. Preservatives clearly serve a public health function in reducing the likelihood of bacterial and fungal infections affecting food. The best known of such bacterial infections is food poisoning from Salmonella contamination. Preservatives reduce biological and chemical degradation and so allow food to have a longer shelf life. However, colours and some of the other agents added to food are of less obvious benefit to the consumer and may be more important to the manufacturer. Enhancing the attractiveness of food is the main reason given for their use but many consumers have become sceptical and have demanded additive-free food or the use of 'natural' additives. Although this may satisfy consumers who believe that natural substances are intrinsically safe, natural products can be as least as toxic as synthetic ones (see Chapter 9). Each 'natural' food additive needs to be assessed individually. As well as

Table 6.1.   Classes of food additives and examples.

Colouring agents	Tartrazine
Anti-oxidants	Butylated hydroxytoluene
Stabilizers	Vegetable gums
Anti-caking agents	Magnesium carbonate
Flavours	Cinnamaldehyde
Preservatives	Sodium nitrate
Emulsifiers	Polyoxyethylene sorbitan fatty esters
Acids/Alkalies	Citric acid
Buffers	Carbonates
Bleaches	Benzoyl peroxide
Propellants	Nitrous oxide
Sweetners	Saccharin
Flavour enhancers	Monosodium glutamate

preservatives other additives may also have a useful function, such as artificial sweeteners which reduce the sugar intake of people with problems such as obesity or diabetes.

As can be appreciated from Table 6.1, food additives comprise a wide range of chemical types from the simple inorganic compounds used as preservatives to the complex organic molecules used as colouring agents and flavours.

In the past, toxic food additives were inadvertently used, such as butter yellow (4-dimethylaminoazobenzene), a dye used to colour butter, which proved to be a carcinogen capable of causing liver tumours in experimental animals.

Clearly food additives have to be tested for toxicity before they can be used and before humans are exposed to them. These tests usually consist of lifetime exposure of experimental animals to the substance at several concentrations, but with the maximum concentration several times greater than that expected to be consumed by humans. However, such testing may not always be predictive as experimental animals may not show the same type of behavioural or immunological effects as does man and absorption, distribution and metabolism can also be different. Also, the administration of relatively large amounts of a substance to experimental animals may lead to accumulation because of saturation of metabolic or excretory pathways. These kinds of problems were encountered with saccharin and clearly make the interpretation of toxicological data difficult. Although the quantities of food additives consumed by humans are very small, their consumption may occur over a lifetime and is chronic although it may be sporadic rather than continuous. This is difficult to simulate in the laboratory animal.

At the present time there is little reliable data on the toxicity of food additives in man but there is much concern on the part of the public and there have been many anecdotal reports of problems relating to food additives, particularly allergic reactions. The incidence of such intolerance to food additives in the population at large is uncertain, most data referring to those patients who have symptoms such as urticaria. In such patients up to half may be responsive to food additives but the figures show wide variation. There may also be cross-reactivity between additives and also with naturally occurring food contaminants such as between salicylates and tartrazine (see below). However certain substances have been removed from the permitted list of additives due to animal data indicating toxicity. One example is that already mentioned, butter yellow. A more recent example is that of the synthetic sweeteners cyclamate and saccharin (see below), both of which suffered from what was interpreted as adverse animal toxicity data and were banned in the USA.

Tartrazine

One well-known example of a food additive, currently in use where there are possible problems in man is the food colour tartrazine, also known as E102 in European countries. This is one of the most widely used colouring agents and also the colour most frequently implicated in intolerance studies especially in pharmaceutical preparations. It is an orange dye used as a colour in drinks such as orange juice but also in a wide variety of other foodstuffs and also in pharmaceutical preparations.

The toxic effects ascribed to tartrazine are the induction of hyperkinetic behaviour or purposeless activity in children, and of urticaria or skin rashes. Hyperkinetic behaviour is difficult to diagnose and distinguish from restlessness which may be due to other factors such as hunger, boredom or inappropriate treatment by adults. The causation of this syndrome by food additives is somewhat controversial as some studies have shown an improvement in behaviour after switching to diets, such as the Feingold diet, which are free from artificial colours and flavours, whereas other studies have shown no improvement. One double-blind cross-over study of 15 hyperkinetic children found some improvement when the Feingold additive-free diet was used. On the one hand, a major change in dietary habits might be expected to cause behavioural changes; on the other hand, another double-blind cross-over study using objective laboratory and classroom observation failed to find any effect of the Feingold diet. Yet, another trial on 22 hyperkinetic children found a statistically significant improvement in the mother's ratings of their children's behaviour but not in objective tests. According to Juhlin, the one study carried out to the most rigorous scientific standards where objective, non-involved observers were used showed no effect of diet on behaviour.

Urticaria due to intake of tartrazine, however, is more widely accepted as an adverse effect and has been demonstrated in a number of studies. There is histamine release and the symptoms are the appearance of red weals on the skin and itching. A number of other food colours and other types of food additive may also cause urticaria and there may be cross reactivity between other colours such as erythrosine and Sunset Yellow. A challenge of patients whose urticaria had improved on a colour-free diet with 0.15 mg of tartrazine resulted in 3 out of 13 developing urticaria within three hours of exposure. Asthma may also be a symptom of hypersensitivity to tartrazine: a study showed that 11 per cent of asthmatics reacted to an orange drink containing colouring agents.

Tartrazine sensitivity is also often related to aspirin intolerance. Indeed, between 10 per cent and 40 per cent of aspirin-sensitive patients respond to tartrazine with reactions ranging from severe asthma to urticaria and mild rhinitis. The mechanism underlying tartrazine sensitivity is unknown but does not seem to involve a reagenic antibody or the prostaglandin synthesis system. A range of antigenic substances in the diet are absorbed from the gastro-intestinal tract but most individuals become immunologically tolerant via a regulatory system which prevents adverse reactions to food constituents and additives. However, some individuals seem predisposed to allergic diseases and do not become immunologically tolerant, hence developing adverse reactions to dietary constituents.

Tartrazine is metabolized by the gut flora giving rise to several metabolites (Figure 2.23) and the urine of animals fed tartrazine has recently been shown to be mutagenic.

Although tartrazine is probably the food colour most commonly implicated in reports of adverse reactions, several others may also cause adverse effects including the 'natural' food colour annatto. Indeed, in one study 26 per cent of patients with chronic urticaria were shown to be responsive to annatto.

Saccharin

This artificial sweetener, first used in the nineteenth century, has been extensively scrutinized over the years and at one stage was banned from use in the USA. As expected of a food additive, saccharin has low acute toxicity, with an LD_{50} of between 5 and 17.7 g kg^{-1} in experimental animals. It is not metabolized and volunteers taking large amounts for several months suffered no ill effects. Two early long-term studies confirmed its safety. Then two studies showed it to be weakly carcinogenic, but these studies have since been criticized as inappropriate. Increased consumption of saccharin and a report showing another sweetener to be carcinogenic prompted further studies to be carried out. In one, saccharin and cyclamate were studied as mixtures with doses up to 2500 mg kg^{-1}. Bladder tumours were observed and as a result cyclamate was banned. Still further studies were carried out but proved inconclusive. Finally, a comprehensive study carried out by the Canadian authorities showed that saccharin could produce bladder tumours in rats and saccharin was suspended from use by the Canadian and US authorities in 1977. In the USA it was banned under the Delaney Clause of the Food, Drug and Cosmetic Act which prohibits the use of any food additive which has been shown to produce cancer in laboratory animals. There was a public outcry against this banning because saccharin was the only general purpose artificial sweetener approved for use and therefore available to diabetics and those with an obesity problem, as well as to other members of the public wishing to reduce their sugar intake. The result was a moratorium on the ban to allow further evidence to be examined. Epidemiological studies mostly showed no increased incidence of bladder tumours but some studies did indicate a slight increase of bladder tumour risk. The absence of detectable metabolism of saccharin after chronic low level dietary exposure and negative mutagenicity data were taken to indicate that saccharin was not a classical electrophilic carcinogen. Therefore, any carcinogenicity was probably due to the unmetabolized parent compound acting by some epigenetic mechanism.

It was found in experimental animals that levels of up to 5 per cent in the diet caused no detectable increase in bladder cancer but levels of 5–7.5 per cent did cause a significant tumour increase. However, pharmacokinetic studies have now shown that the plasma clearance of saccharin is saturated at the higher exposure level, giving higher tissue concentrations than would be predicted from a linear extrapolation of data from lower dose studies. Consequently, such high-level exposure in animals may be inappropriate as regards normal human exposure. The saccharin case illustrates the wider social aspects as well as the scientific considerations involved with toxicology. There are value judgements to be made and risk must be balanced against benefit. These issues will be addressed in the final chapter.

Food Contaminants

As well as intentional food additives, foodstuffs may also contain contaminants. These might be toxic bacterial or fungal products, toxic degradation products from food constituents, such as pyrolysis products resulting from cooking, or they might be substances inadvertently added to the food. There is now great interest in toxic and especially carcinogenic compounds produced as a result of cooking such as the mutagenic compounds Trp 1 and Trp 2, and carcinogenic nitroso compounds produced from dietary amines.

Two examples of naturally occurring but toxic food contaminants are botulinum toxin and aflatoxin. Botulism will only be briefly discussed here as it is covered in more detail in Chapter 9 under natural products.

Botulism

Botulism is the syndrome caused by botulinum toxin from the bacterium *Clostridium botulinum*. This anaerobic bacterium may contaminate tinned or bottled food and the toxin is extremely potent. Heating destroys the toxin.

Aflatoxin

The aflatoxins are a group of mycotoxins produced by the mould *Aspergillus flavus*. This mould may grow on foodstuffs such as damp peanuts and stored crops, particularly under hot, humid conditions, and the resulting contamination can be a serious problem in some tropical countries. Tainted crops are difficult to sell to countries such as the USA and UK which have strict criteria on levels of mycotoxins. Consequently, the tainted crops may then be sold within the poorer producing country or may find their way to famine victims as part of the relief effort.

Animals fed on meal derived from contaminated feed such as peanuts may develop tumours. The toxins were in fact discovered as a result of the loss of turkeys suffering liver damage after being given mouldy feed. Also, traces of aflatoxin have been detected in peanut butter, especially that made from peanuts not treated with chemicals to prevent mould growth and consequently sold in health food shops labelled as 'natural'.

Aflatoxin B_1 is a very potent liver carcinogen and hepatotoxin; a level of 1 ppb in the diet may be sufficient to cause liver tumours. Levels of aflatoxin in the diet are higher (ppm as opposed to ppb) in Africa than in other parts of the world and this explains the higher incidence of liver cancer in certain parts of Africa. The mechanism of toxicity of aflatoxin B_1 involves metabolism to a chemically reactive intermediate (an epoxide) which binds covalently to protein but which also interacts with nucleic acids. This chemically reactive intermediate may be responsible for both the liver necrosis and the liver tumours.

Ptaquiloside

See Chapter 9 for a discussion of this naturally occuring carcinogen found in edible bracken fern shoots.

The Spanish Oil Syndrome

Non-natural substances may also sometimes contaminate food and there have been several examples of this such as Epping jaundice which has already been mentioned in chapter 5. A more recent and tragic example of this was the contamination of cooking oil in Spain.

In May 1981 an unusual outbreak of a pulmonary disease was reported around Madrid. The unusual syndrome included severe pulmonary oedema which was not prolonged, exanthema and eosinophilia. Overall there were more than 20 000 cases of the syndrome and 351 fatalities (Figure 6.1). A toxic substance was suspected and finally a connection was established between the disease and the use of cheap cooking oil. Action by the Spanish Government to replace the oil with pure olive oil decreased the numbers of cases reported. There was a correlation between the consumption of cheap oil, especially that sold by certain salesmen, and the development of the syndrome.

The disease appeared after a latent period of at least 1–2 weeks, longer in some cases, and an apparent dose-response relationship was noted in one report. However, the association between the intake of oil and the syndrome is circumstantial as the effects have not been reproduced in experimental animals and the precise causative agent has not been identified. The syndrome had an acute phase with mainly acute pulmonary interstitial oedema, and a chronic phase which was mainly neuromuscular with muscular atrophy, skin lesions and weight loss. Vasculitis was also observed which affected many blood vessels.

SPAIN'S POISON OIL SCANDAL

THE SUNDAY TIMES, 23 AUGUST 1981

Figure 6.1. A headline reporting the disaster which followed the use of rape-seed oil contaminated with aniline as a substitute for olive oil in Spain in 1981.
From *The Sunday Times*, August 23 1981, with permission.

The toxic oil was rape-seed oil which had been denatured by the addition of aniline, as required by law in Spain for imported rape seed oil so that it cannot be used for cooking. However, refining of this oil was undertaken and the resulting oil sold as suitable for human consumption. This had been practised previously without the toxic effects being seen, and consequently it seems that the particular batch of oil responsible for the syndrome may have been refined differently or was different in some other way. It was mixed with other oils in some cases and so may have become contaminated. Identifying the toxic constituents so far has not been possible. The failure to understand the mechanism underlying this major public health disaster highlights the difficulties of studying food additive/contaminant problems. These are often due to factors beyond the control of the toxicologist. In this case, the problem of obtaining samples of oil reliably associated with the syndrome and the absence of an animal model have greatly hampered the research.

This tragedy also illustrates how a large number of people may be affected by a toxic contaminant in a foodstuff. A more subtle toxic reaction to a food additive than the one described here could affect many more people before it was detected.

Questions

1. Write short notes on the toxicological aspects of the following:

   (a) aflatoxin;
   (b) ptaquiloside;
   (c) botulinum toxin.

2. What particular problems are associated with the safety evaluation of food additives? Illustrate your answer with reference to saccharin.

Bibliography

Ballantyne, B., Marrs, T. and Turner, P. (1993) (Eds) *General and Applied Toxicology*, Basingstoke, UK: Macmillan.

Conning, D. M. (1993) Toxicology of Food and Food Additives, In: *General and Applied Toxicology*, Ballantyne, B., Marrs, T. and Turner, P. (Eds), Basingstoke, UK: Macmillan.

Hanssen, M. and Marsden, J. (1984) *E for Additives*, Wellingborough: Thorsons.

Juhlin, L. (1983) Intolerance to food and drug additives, in *Allergic Reactions to Drugs*, de Weck, A. L. and Bundgaard, H. (Eds) Berlin: Springer Verlag.

Lin, J-K. and Ho, Y-S. (1994) Hepatotoxic Actions of Dietary Amines. *Toxicology and Ecotoxicology News*, **1**, 82–87.

Miller, K. and Nicklin, S. (1984) Adverse reactions to food additives and colours, in *Developments in Food Colours*, vol. 2, Walford, J. (Ed.), Amsterdam: Elsevier Applied Science.

Miller, S. A. (1991) Food Additives and Contaminants, in *Cassarett and Doull's Toxicology*, Amdur, M. O., Doull, J. and Klaassen, C. (Eds) 4th edition, New York: Pergamon Press.

NAS (1978) Saccharin: Technical Assessment of Risks and Benefits, Report No. 1, Washington, DC: Committee for a Study on Saccharin and Food Safety Policy.

Rechcigl, M. (Ed.) (1983) *Handbook of Naturally Occurring Food Toxicants*, Boca Raton: CRC Press.

World Health Organisation (1984) Toxic Oil Syndrome, Report on a WHO Meeting, Madrid 1983, Copenhagen: WHO.

Chapter 7

Pesticides

Introduction

Pesticides are substances which have been designed or chosen for selective toxicity to certain organisms. Although their toxicity *is* selective, they are often also toxic to other species although usually to a lesser degree. As well as being of interest in terms of their mode of action they are of concern to toxicologists for two reasons: (1) they may be toxic to man either in acute poisonings or after chronic exposure; and (2) they have toxic effects on some non-target organisms in the environment. This latter point was highlighted in 1963 by Rachel Carson in her book *Silent Spring*.

Human poisonings from accidental exposure to pesticides have occurred since they were first used and in some cases many people have been poisoned, sometimes fatally in single incidents. Many of these cases have been due to accidental contamination of food with pesticides or their inappropriate use (Table 7.1). For example, the use of organic mercury fungicides to treat seed grain which is then used to feed animals has resulted in several mass poisonings of humans. Occupational poisoning has also occurred in agricultural workers through accidental contamination or inappropriate use. The careless use of pesticides, such as spraying without adequate protection, may also lead to exposure of the operator.

Chronic toxicity due to the pesticides present in our environment is more difficult to identify although with the development of improved analytical techniques the detection of residues has become easier. Such techniques have shown that most people in the Western World are indeed exposed to and in many cases contaminated with, certain pesticides. However, pesticides have become a very important part of our society especially in terms of agricultural economics and, although their use may be curtailed in some instances, it is unlikely to be completely halted when risk/benefit considerations are made.

Pesticides can be divided into several groups, such as insecticides, fungicides, herbicides and rodenticides, depending on the target organism. Those that have been specifically designed for a purpose often utilize a particular biological, metabolic or other feature of the target species, but unfortunately such features are rarely entirely unique to that species so other similar species may also be affected. A simple example of selective toxicity in a pesticide is

Table 7.1. Mass poisonings due to pesticides.

Pesticide involved	Material contaminated	Number affected	(died)	Location
Endrin	Flour	159	(0)	Wales
Endrin	Four	691	(24)	Qatar
Parathion	Flour	600	(88)	Colombia
Parathion	Sugar	300	(17)	Mexico
Hexachlorobenzene	Seed grain	>3000	(3–11%)	Turkey
Organic mercury	Seed grain	321	(35)	Iraq
Pentachlorophenol	Nursery linens	20	(2)	USA

Source: *Report of the Secretary's Commission on Pesticides and Their Relationship to Environmental Health*, (Washington, DC: US Governmental Printing Office, 1969).

the use of warfarin as a rodenticide. This depends on the lack of the vomit reflex in rats so that they are unable to vomit after ingesting the poison.

Other pesticides depend on more sophisticated biochemical differences. For example, the insecticide malathion is metabolized by hydrolysis in mammals to yield the acidic metabolite, which is readily excreted (Figure 2.20). In insects, however, the preferred metabolic route is oxidation to yield malaoxon which is toxic by inhibition of cholinesterase (see below). Although pesticides may all be perceived by the general public as equally hazardous to man, they vary in their toxicity to mammals, and other non target wildlife, and in their effects on the environment.

Some examples of the major pesticide types are as follows:

Insecticides: Organophosphorus compounds, carbamate and organo-chlorine compounds. Natural products such as pyrethrins.
Herbicides: Chlorophenoxy compounds, dinitrophenols, bipyridyls, carbamates, triazines, substituted ureas, aromatic amides.
Fungicides: alkyl mercury compounds, chlorinated hydrocarbons, dialkyldithiocarbamates, organotin compounds.
Rodenticides: inorganic agents, natural products, fluorinated aliphatics, α-naphthylthiourea.

It is clear from this list that pesticides comprise a wide range of chemical types and their modes of action will be very different. However, their toxicity to man and other mammals may be due to a different mechanism from their pesticidal action.

We will now consider some toxicologically important examples of pesticides.

DDT

Perhaps the best known organochlorine insecticide is DDT, (dichloro-diphenyl-trichloroethane; Figure 7.1). It was introduced in 1945 for the control of malarial mosquitoes and was extremely successful, being a major

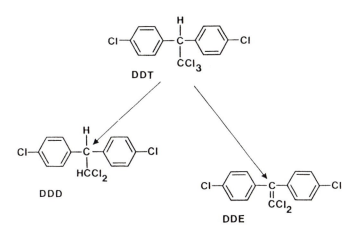

Figure 7.1. Two of the pathways of metabolism of the insecticide dichloro-diphenyl-trichloroethane (DDT).

factor in the reduction in malaria after the Second World War. DDT is a contact poison which is highly potent against the insect nervous system but is relatively non-toxic to man. A dose of at least 10 mg kg^{-1} is required for toxic effects to occur in man and no human fatalities have been reported. Indeed human volunteers were induced to take 0.5 mg kg^{-1} (35 mg) daily for over a year and there was no demonstrable toxicity. Although some reports have suggested association between chronic disease and DDT, no causal relationship has been found and other reports have not found such associations. Large doses cause tremors, hyperexcitability and convulsions, paresthesias, irritability and dizziness. In experimental animals liver damage occurs after single large doses and hypertrophy and other histological changes in liver have been reported after chronic exposure. Toxic effects seem mainly to involve the nervous system in mammals as in insects. The mechanism of action is unknown but the primary site of action is thought to be sensory; motor nerve fibres and the motor cortex are possible targets. DDT may alter transport of Na$^+$ and K$^+$ across nerve membranes perhaps by interfering with the energy metabolism required for this transport.

DDT is chemically stable, highly insoluble in water, but soluble in body fat and is consequently very persistent in biological systems and the environment (Table 7.2). It is poorly absorbed through the skin and is metabolized in animals by a number of routes (Figure 7.1) but the metabolite DDE is more persistent than the parent compound (Table 7.2). There are other metabolites

Table 7.2. Persistence of the insecticide DDT and its metabolites.

Compound	Half-life in pigeon (days)	Half-life in soil (yrs)
DDT	28	2.5–5
DDD	23	
DDE	250	

such as an acidic derivative which is more water-soluble but the conversion to these is slow and does not involve major routes. There are also microbial and environmental degradation to other metabolites.

It is because of this persistence, that DDT levels in the environment have been increasing ever since it was first used. Furthermore, the DDT concentration in some of the exposed organisms increases at each higher trophic level of the food chain (see Chapter 8). For example, small organisms such as plankton or daphnia absorb DDT passively or via filter feeding from river or lake water and this enters their body fat. The concentration in the tissues of these organisms may be several hundred or thousand fold greater than the concentration in the surrounding water. Then, either insects or small fish eat these small organisms and the DDT is transferred to their fat tissue (Table 7.3). These small organisms are in turn eaten by still larger organisms and so on up the food chain. As DDT is fat soluble it remains in the organism and is then transferred into the fat of the predator or animal at the top of the food chain which may be man. The result is that relatively high concentrations of DDT can occur in those animals at the top of the food chain by a continuous process of amplification or biomagnification despite the fact that the initial concentration of DDT in the water is low. This is illustrated by the following example: in one area of California plankton were found to contain 4 ppm of DDT, while the bass found in the same area contained 138 ppm and the grebes feeding on them 1500 ppm. So what seems to be a negligible concentration of DDT in the river or lake water or at the bottom of a food chain may be biologically very significant at the top. Toxic concentrations of DDT appear to affect birds and fish particularly in the production of eggs. It can be shown, for example, that there is a relationship between shell thickness and DDE concentration in birds of prey such as the kestrel (Figure 7.2).

In man, as in other animals exposed to DDT, most is located in the body fat. The concentration in fat is proportional to the intake, reaching a plateau with a half-life of around six months. The estimated intake for humans in USA was around 35 mg year^{-1} in 1969 but the level in food is declining as is the amount in human fat. The acceptable yearly intake for humans as given by the FAO/WHO guidelines is 255 mg year^{-1}. The DDT either comes from eating food of animal origin where the animal itself or another lower in the food chain has been exposed, or from vegetables or fruit which have been sprayed or otherwise contaminated.

The DDT in fat does not appear to be harmful to animals, however, and there is no correlation between adipose tissue levels and signs of poisoning.

Table 7.3. Example of a food chain.

Organism	Tropic Level
Pine trees	1st Producers
Aphids	2nd Herbivores
Spiders	3rd Insectivores
Tits and Warblers	4th Insectivores
Hawks	5th Carnivores

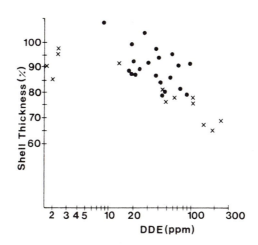

Figure 7.2. The relationship between shell thickness and residues of the DDT metabolite DDE. The data is from kestrel eggs collected in Ithaca, New York in 1970 (●) or experimentally induced with dietary DDE (X). The data is the mean clutch thickness expressed as percent of control egg thickness collected before DDT use. Data from Lincer, J. L. (1975), *Journal of Applied Ecology*, **12**, 781.

It is the concentration circulating in the blood which is more relevant to the toxic effects, and more particularly the level in the brain. However, if there is a reduction of the fat content of the body, the blood level will rise. Experiments with rats have shown that this increase in blood level can lead to toxicity. It has been found recently that bats in the southern USA have high levels of DDT even though it is no longer used. This is probably because the bats eat large quantities of insects and there is sufficient residual DDT in the environment for it to appear in food chains. In a particular species of bat this has been a problem because the DDT is passed via the milk to young bats and this then enters their fat tissues. When the bats go on mass long distance-migration, they start to mobilize this fat and so their blood levels of DDT increase until they become sufficient to cause toxicity and death.

Human milk may also contain DDT and as with other food chains there is a concentration effect. For example, lactating mothers exposed to 0.0005 mg kg^{-1} day^{-1} were found to produce milk containing 0.08 ppm DDT, hence their infants were exposed to 0.0112 mg kg^{-1} day^{-1}, an exposure some twenty times greater than the mothers.

There is no real evidence that DDT under such chronic exposure conditions is overtly toxic in man although there is some evidence that it is carcinogenic in mice. Consequently continuous exposure to low levels of DDT may constitute a long-term hazard. Chronic exposure to DDT does lead to induction of the microsomal enzymes involved in the metabolism of foreign compounds. It may be this effect that causes the hormonal imbalance seen in birds, as some hormones are also metabolized by the microsomal enzymes.

Most other organochlorine insecticides such as heptachlor, gamma-HCH, dieldrin and aldrin, have similar problems of persistence to DDT.

Organophosphorus Compounds

The use of organochlorine insecticides has decreased recently because of their persistence and because of fears about their long-term effects. The case against DDT is mainly due to its environmental impact on wildlife rather than its toxicity to man, which seems to be low. However, the organophosphorus compounds which have replaced the organochlorine type of insecticide are often more toxic to mammals (maybe as much as one hundred times more toxic) if less persistent. For example, organophosphorus compounds are the major cause of poisoning in agricultural workers in California.

There are many organophosphorus compounds now used as insecticides and their mode of action and toxicity is similar. As already indicated organophosphorus compounds are more toxic and have been responsible for more human deaths and illness than the organochlorine type of pesticide. Parathion, first synthesized in 1944 (Figure 7.3), is one widely used organophosphorus insecticide which has featured in a number of documented mass human poisonings (Table 7.1) and probably in many isolated incidents. Parathion has high mammalian toxicity and consequently it has been superseded by other less toxic organophosphorus compounds for certain uses. One such insecticide is malathion (Figure 2.20) which is more selective in its toxicity mainly because of differences in its metabolism between mammals and insects. However, the effects of organophosphorus compounds are qualitatively similar and can be considered collectively.

Poisoning with organophosphorus compounds is an example of an exaggerated pharmacological effect rather than of direct toxic action and the toxicity may be either cumulative following chronic exposure or acute after a single exposure. The toxic effects are due to the inhibition of cholinesterase enzymes, in particular acetylcholinesterase, by the organophosphate. This enzyme is responsible for the hydrolysis of acetylcholine to choline and acetate (Figure 7.4) which effectively terminates the action of acetylcholine as a chemical transmitter of nerve impulses at synaptic nerve endings. The result of the inhibition by organophosphorus compounds is a build up of acetylcholine and so excessive stimulation of the nerve. Depending on the particular organophosphorus compound the inhibition may be reversible or irreversible. The acetylcholinesterases in different tissues such as plasma and nerves are different and so are not equally inhibited by organophosphorus compounds. There are degrees of inhibition of the total body acetylcholinesterase; in mammals a level of 50 per cent inhibition leads to toxic effects and 80–90 per

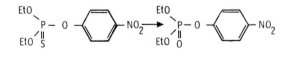

Parathion   Paraoxon

Figure 7.3. The oxidative metabolism of the insecticide parathion.
From Timbrell, J. A., *Principles of Biochemical Toxicology*, Taylor & Francis, London, 1991.

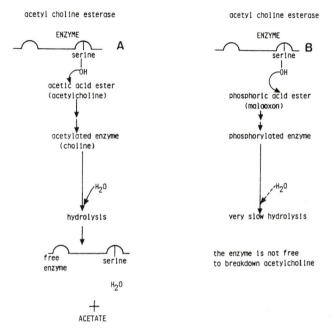

Figure 7.4. The mechanisms of hydrolysis of acetylcholine by acetylcholinesterase (A) and the interaction of the malathion metabolite malaoxon with the enzyme (B).

cent inhibition will be lethal. The mechanism of toxicity of organophosphorus compounds relies on their similarity to the normal substrate acetylcholine (Figure 7.4). Thus, the organophosphorus compound is also a substrate for the enzyme but unlike acetylcholine, the product remains bound to the active site and the resulting complex may be only slowly hydrolyzed, if at all. With those organophosphorus compounds causing irreversible inhibition, resynthesis of the enzyme is necessary.

Malathion itself is not a substrate for cholinesterases but requires metabolism to malaoxon. This takes place readily in insects but in mammals hydrolysis is the preferred route and this leads to a readily excreted diacid (Figure 2.20). This is the basis of the selective toxicity.

The toxic effects of organophosphorus compounds centre around the excessive cholinergic stimulation with death occurring a a result of neuro-muscular paralysis and central depression. Some organophosphorus compounds may also cause damage to the peripheral nerves but this delayed neurotoxic effect is believed to be caused by a different mechanism.

Paraquat

The examples mentioned so far have been insecticides which, as a group, are probably more important than other pesticides in terms of human and environmental toxicity. However, one particular herbicide is of particular importance and notoriety in terms of human toxicology. This is paraquat (Figure 7.5) which, during the twenty years of its use, has featured in several hundred cases of fatal human poisoning. Unlike the organophosphorus compounds, however, this has not been the result of accidental contamination of food and unlike the organochlorines there has been no particular environmental impact. Paraquat poisoning has mainly been the result of deliberate ingestion, usually orally, for suicide or murder with a few cases of accidental direct ingestion. Paraquat is a contact herbicide which binds very strongly to soil. Consequently it does not leach out of soil after being sprayed onto plants and does not have an environmental effect either on other plants or animals. Paraquat kills the plant by interfering with photosynthesis and its toxicity to animals may have some similarities at the biochemical level. When ingested by humans paraquat is usually fatal but even if it is not it may cause serious lung and kidney damage. The lung is the target organ because it *selectively* accumulates paraquat and consequently the concentration in the alveolar type I and II lung cells reaches sufficient levels to cause toxic effects in those cells. The concentration in the lungs reaches a level several times that in the plasma and the paraquat is retained in the lung even when the plasma concentration is falling. Paraquat is taken up by the lung because of a structural similarity with diamines and polyamines, such as putrescine, spermine and spermidine (Figure 7.5). The presence of two nitrogens in paraquat, with a particular intramolecular distance, enables paraquat, but not the herbicide diquat, to be taken up by a selective active transport system in the lung for which polyamines are the normal substrate. The only other organ with an uptake system for polyamines is the brain which does not seem to accumulate paraquat.

Paraquat is believed to cause toxicity via its free radical form which is stable and results from an enzyme-mediated, one electron reduction which requires NADPH (Figure 7.6). In the presence of oxygen this generates superoxide anion and the paraquat cation reforms. This redox cycling continues to produce superoxide and deplete NADPH. The superoxide can lead to the production of hydrogen peroxide and hydroxyl radicals. Hydroxyl radicals are highly reactive and can cause lipid peroxidation which in turn causes further metabolic disruption. The presence of oxygen in the lungs is clearly an important factor in the pathogenesis of the lung lesion. The toxicity to the

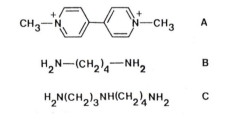

Figure 7.5. The structure of the herbicide paraquat (A), and the polyamines putrescine (B) and spermine (C)

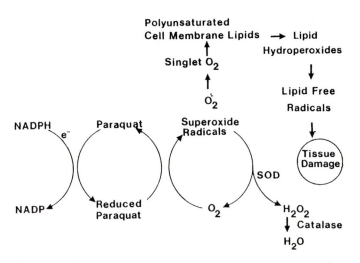

Figure 7.6. The proposed mechanism for the lung toxicity of paraquat. SOD is the enzyme superoxide dismutase.
Adapted from Data from Vale, J. A. and Meredith, T. J., Paraquat Poisoning, pp. 135–141, Figure 21.2 in *Poisoning-Diagnosis and Treatment*, Vale, J. A. and Meredith, T. J., (Eds) Update Books, London, 1981.

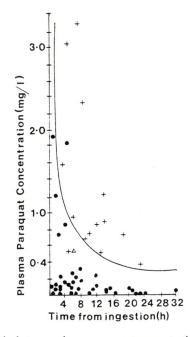

Figure 7.7. The relationship between plasma paraquat concentration and the outcome of the poisoning, death (+) or survival (•). ∆ is an aspiration death.
Data from Vale, J. A. and Meredith, T. J., Paraquat Poisoning, pp. 135–141, Figure 21.4 in *Poisoning-Diagnosis and Treatment*, Vale, J. A. and Meredith, T. J., (Eds) Update Books, London, 1981.

lungs is a direct result of the distribution of paraquat as the active uptake into lung cells gives rise to the relatively high and toxic concentration.

Paraquat causes a progressive fibrosis of the lungs and also damages the kidneys; once absorbed there is no antidote. The only treatments available are either an attempt to limit absorption by oral administration of substances such as Fullers Earth which adsorb paraquat or the use of haemodialysis or haemoperfusion to rid the blood of the paraquat. After the paraquat has accumulated in the lungs, however, there is no effective treatment currently available.

Paraquat has been used on many occasions for suicide and parasuicide attempts but unfortunately for the victim death is slow and painful, occurring over a period of a several days to a week or more with the progressive fibrosis of the lung leading to eventual suffocation. The prognosis is usually bad and the plasma level of paraquat indicates the likely outcome (Figure 7.7).

Fluoroacetate

Monofluoroacetate is an interesting example of a pesticide which is also a natural product. This compound is highly toxic by virtue of its very specific blockade of Krebs (tricarboxylic acid) cycle. Fluoroacetate is a pseudo-substrate and is successfully incorporated into Krebs cycle as fluoroacetyl CoA. The fluorocitrate produced will bind to the enzyme aconitase, but after binding the pseudosubstrate, the enzyme cannot remove the fluorine atom and so the enzyme is blocked. Therefore, Krebs cycle is unable to function and the cell and organism dies through lack of metabolic intermediates and energy.

Fluoroacetate is found naturally in some plants in Australia, Africa and South America. Some indigenous animals in Australia, especially the skink and emu have developed tolerance. However, introduced and unadapted animals, such as rats, mice, cats and dogs and those living outside the areas where fluoroacetate producing plants grow, are more susceptible to fluoroacetate toxicity (see Twigg and King, 1991). This is a example of what has been termed 'chemical warfare' between plants and animals. The plants produce such toxic substances to stop animals eating them. However, fluoroacetate is also used as a pesticide for example in New Zealand, where it is known as 1080 and is used to kill possums which have become pests.

Questions

1. Contrast the toxicology of organochlorine insecticides such as DDT and the organophosphorus type such as parathion.
2. Discuss the toxicology of paraquat and in particular explain the mechanism underlying the specific organ damage.
3. Explain what is meant by the term 'selective toxicity'. Illustrate your answer with specific examples.

Bibliography

Echobichon, D. J. (1991) Toxic Effects of Pesticides, in *Cassarett and Doull's Toxicology*, Amdur, M. O., Doull, J. and Klaassen, C. (Eds), 4th edition, New York: Pergamon Press.

Hayes, W. J. (1975) *Toxicology of Pesticides*, Baltimore: Waverley Press.

Hayes, W. J. (1982) *Pesticides Studied in Man*, Baltimore: Williams and Wilkins.

Marrs, T. C. (1993) Toxicology of Pesticides, in Ballantyne, B., Marrs, T. and Turner, P. (Eds) *General and Applied Toxicology*, Basingstoke, UK: Macmillan.

Matsumura, F. (1975), *Toxicology of Insecticides*, New York: Plenum Press.

Twigg, L. E. and King, D. R. (1991) The impact of fluoroacetate-bearing vegetation on native Australian fauna: a review. OIKOS 61: 412–430.

Chapter 8

Environmental Pollutants

Introduction

Pollution of our environment has become an increasing problem over the last century with the development of industry and agriculture and with the increase in population. That is not to say that pollution did not exist before the nineteenth century, indeed there was legislation enacted in Britain during the thirteenth century to control smoke from household fires in London. However, pollution on the current scale started during the Industrial Revolution. Nineteenth-century factories used coal for fuel and in certain processes, and consequently smoke was a major pollutant. Blast furnaces and chemical plants added other fumes and other types of noxious substance. As many industrial processes used water for power, as part of the process, or in some other way, factories were often sited near rivers and effluent was discharged into them. In this way both the atmosphere and rivers became polluted. More recently the land has also become polluted from agricultural use of fertilizers and pesticides, as well as from the dumping of toxic wastes from factories and industrial processes. Consequently air, water and the earth have all suffered pollution and we may divide environmental pollution into these categories.

Despite the appalling working and living conditions which existed during the Industrial Revolution in parts of Britain during the nineteenth century and in heavily industrialized areas in other European countries and the USA, it was not until the twentieth century that a serious attempt was made to curb pollution. One event which precipitated this was the 'great smog' in London in the winter of 1952. A combination of weather conditions and smoke from domestic coal fires, factories and power stations resulted in a thick smog which contributed to the deaths of over four thousand people (Figure 8.1).

At around the same time the River Thames was found to be so highly polluted that fish, particularly salmon, could not live in the lower parts of the river. This was as a result of industrial processes and other processes dumping effluent into the river. The same was true in some other cities in the UK and in other industrial countries.

In Britain, as a result of the smog, the Clean Air Act was passed which led to a reduction in the production of smoke in cities. Other legislation concerned with pollution of rivers allowed the gradual clean-up of the Thames. Now

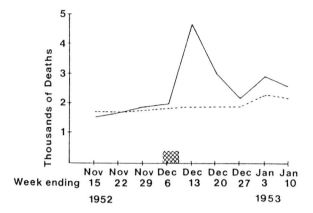

Figure 8.1. Deaths associated with the London 'fog' of December 1952. The solid curve shows the number of weekly deaths in Greater London before and after the 'fog' whereas the dotted line shows the average number of deaths for the preceding 5 years. The hatched area shows the dates of the 'fog'.
Data from Goldsmith, J. R. in *Air Pollution*, Vol. 1. Chapter 10, pp. 335–386, Figure 1. Ed. A. C. Stern, NY: Academic Press, 1962.

smogs in London no longer occur and there are salmon swimming in the Thames. This has taken many years, however, and in other parts of Britain, as in some other countries, clean-up of the environment has not always been so successful. Air pollution from coal-burning power stations still occurs and it is now recognized that this pollution travels many hundreds of miles from countries such as Britain to Norway, Sweden and Germany, and from the USA to Canada. In these countries the air pollutants and acid rain (see page 108) cause damage to trees and other plant life and also to fish and other aquatic organisms. This illustrates that pollution is an international rather than a purely national problem.

Pollution of the environment is usually a continuous, deliberate process although industrial and other accidents may also contribute to environmental pollution in an acute rather than chronic manner. Let us consider some examples of environmental pollution.

Air Pollution

The study of air pollution involves many disciplines ranging from chemistry, engineering, epidemiology, zoology, botany, ecology, toxicology and meteorology to economics and politics. It is not a new phenomenon although it has only relatively recently become of such importance.

The most visible form of air pollution is of course smoke but this contains many constituents depending on the source and is accompanied by various potentially toxic gases. The burning of the fossil fuels coal and oil as well as certain industrial processes give rise to the gases sulphur dioxide, carbon dioxide, carbon monoxide and nitrogen oxides, and perhaps hydrogen sulphide, volatile hydrocarbons, and particulate matter such as carbon and ash. In Britain these amount to millions of tonnes per year; sulphur dioxide from burning fuel amounts to at least 4 million tonnes discharged into the atmosphere every year. In the USA the five major pollutants which amount to 98 per cent of all the air pollution are carbon monoxide (52 per cent), sulphur oxides (18 per cent), hydrocarbons (12 per cent), particulates (10 per cent) and nitrogen oxides (6 per cent). These air pollutants arise from the combustion of fuels in power stations and domestically, from car exhausts, from industrial processes, and from waste disposal.

The composition and dispersion of air pollutants may also be influenced by climatic conditions and can lead to 'smog'. Originally this term was coined to describe the combination of fog and smoke which hung over industrial cities under damp atmospheric conditions but it now also includes air pollution from car exhausts which has been modified by climatic conditions.

There are in fact two types of smog. (1) Reducing smog which has a high level of particulates and sulphur dioxide and comes from coal burning in particular. It results from a combination of incomplete combustion, fog and cool temperatures. (2) Photochemical-oxidant smog, for which Los Angeles is notorious, has a high concentration of ozone, nitrogen oxides and hydrocarbons. This is an oxidizing pollutant mixture arising particularly from the interaction of the constituents of car exhausts in bright sunlight. Meteorologic inversion, as occurs in the Los Angeles basin, not only promotes this interaction but also traps the pollutants near the ground. The constituents of air pollution may in turn be altered in the atmosphere. For example, hydrogen sulphide and nitrogen dioxide may be oxidized to sulphuric and nitric acids respectively.

Ozone arises from a cyclic reaction between nitrogen dioxide and oxygen, with ultraviolet light and hydrocarbons as necessary catalysts:

$$NO_2 \xrightarrow{uv} NO + O$$
$$O_2 + O \rightarrow O_3$$
$$O_3 + NO \rightarrow NO_2 + O_2$$

What are the effects of all these pollutants on the health of man and the animals and plants in the environment?

Some of the acute effects on human health are known from several episodes which have occurred within the last 50 years. The three major episodes which have led to increased human mortality and morbidity were in the Meuse Valley in Belgium (1930), in Donora, Pennsylvania (1948), and in London (1952). In each case the area was heavily polluted and the same meteorological conditions (inversion) prevailed which allowed a stagnant mass of polluted air to accumulate and the pollution level to rise.

Sixty-five people died in Belgium and twenty in Donora. *Four thousand* deaths in London were attributed to the smog (Figure 8.1). These deaths were mainly in elderly people who already had respiratory or cardiac disease. After the smog in Belgium it had been predicted that a similar occurrence in London would led to 3200 extra deaths. In fact there were 4000. On the worst day of the smog, the daily average pollutant levels were: sulphur dioxide 1.34 ppm and smoke 4.5 mg m^{-3}. Another London smog in 1962 resulted in 400 extra deaths. It has been estimated that a sulphur dioxide level of 0.25 ppm and a smoke level of 0.75 mg m^{-3} will produce an increase in mortality over the normal rate. Epidemiological studies of human populations have shown a higher incidence of pulmonary and cardiovascular disease in association with smog. Air pollution is believed to be a factor in lung cancer, the incidence of which is higher in urban areas but there are many unknown and possibly confounding factors. Some correlation has also been detected between certain other diseases, such as heart disease, with pollution levels. Chronic air pollution certainly aggravates existing respiratory diseases including the common cold and may even be a contributory factor. Filtration of air gives relief to some susceptible individuals. One early study in Britain showed a striking correlation between levels of certain pollutants (the reducing type) and the level of discomfort of patients with chronic bronchitis. It was estimated that the levels of smoke and sulphur dioxide needed to be below 0.25 mg m^{-3} and 0.19 ppm respectively for there to be no response. Indeed, the mortality from chronic bronchitis is correlated with the amount of sulphur dioxide and dust levels.

There is, however, less data on the effects of photochemical-oxidant pollution on human health. One study examined the performance of an athletic team in Los Angeles in the USA over several seasons and monitored photochemical-oxidant pollutant levels. There was a striking correlation between the level of oxidizing pollutants in the air and a decrease in performance, with effects demonstrated at a level as low as 0.1 ppm. The mean oxidant level in Los Angeles at this time exceeded 0.1 ppm and the maximum hourly level reached 0.6 ppm at certain times. Lung function as measured by forced expiratory volume is measurably reduced in people living in polluted areas but such data do not indicate which pollutant is responsible and other factors may be equally important.

Experimental exposure of animals or human volunteers to individual pollutants shows toxic effects on pulmonary airways such as constriction and, hence, increased resistance, but synergistic effects occur between pollutants when they are present in mixtures. For example, the reaction between sulphur dioxide, water and ozone to give sulphuric acid is facilitated by the presence of hydrocarbons and particulates. Sulphur dioxide is an irritant but its lethal concentration is far greater than the amount normally encountered in air pollution. Levels of sulphur dioxide greater than 0.05 ppm have been reputed to cause an increased incidence of respiratory illness and chronic exposure to levels above 0.2 ppm increased mortality. Exposure to levels of 1–5 ppm gives rise to acute discomfort. Smoke has a synergistic effect on sulphur dioxide toxicity so that the combination has a greater effect than either individual constituent.

Nitrogen dioxide and ozone are more toxic than sulphur dioxide and are deep lung irritants. Nitrogen oxides arise from car exhaust and other sources and cause respiratory symptoms at concentrations of 5–10 ppm. The levels of nitrogen oxides in Los Angeles average 0.7 ppm. Ozone causes damage to sensitive plants and affects humans suffering from asthma at levels of 50 ppb, yet in July 1976 concentrations of 260 ppb of ozone were measured in Britain and these levels were maintained for a week. The permitted level of ozone in factories is 80 ppb.

Carbon monoxide is another constituent of pollution, especially that derived from car exhausts. Although the chronic toxic effects of carbon monoxide are uncertain, the acute effects are well known (see Chapter 10). Carbon monoxide is very toxic, binding avidly to haemoglobin in competition with oxygen so as to reduce the ability of the blood to supply oxygen to the tissues. This will cause brain damage and death at high levels of blood saturation. It has been suggested that chronic exposure to carbon monoxide may cause heart damage resulting from tissue anoxia. Changes in blood pressure, pulse rate and cardiac output occur after 30 per cent saturation of blood with carbon monoxide, which is achieved at an ambient concentration of 75 ppm. The urban air concentration may be around 10–20 ppm resulting in about 4–8 per cent saturation. However, exposure levels as high as 100 ppm may be experienced in some circumstances such as by traffic policemen. These concentrations cause dizziness, headache and lassitude. Levels of 120 ppm for one hour or 30 ppm for eight hours are considered serious in the USA. Carbon monoxide is also present in cigarette smoke and heavy smoking may result in a level of more than 7 per cent carboxyhaemoglobin in the blood of the smoker. It is not clear whether exposure to carbon monoxide in the environment over the long term is a significant health hazard although it is believed to be an important factor in the cardiovascular effects of smoking. A positive correlation has been shown between carbon monoxide levels and myocardial infarction in Los Angeles but there were other confounding factors. Some individuals, however, such as those with anaemia who have low blood haemoglobin, are more sensitive to carbon monoxide than normal healthy people.

Pollution from power stations and especially car exhausts also contains hydrocarbons and these may be carcinogenic or have other toxic effects. The particulates present in smoke may become deposited in the lungs but this depends on the particle size as already described in Chapter 2. However, conclusive data on the effects of these pollutants on human health are not available. There are so many environmental factors which may adversely affect human health that attributing morbidity to a particular air pollutant is difficult.

Particulates

As well as airborne gases such as nitrogen oxides and substances such as lead, there are also particles present in the air we breathe. There is currently much concern about particular sized small particles, the so called PM10. These are particles which are less than 10 μm in diameter derived from cars and other vehicles. The particles vary in chemical composition but may simply be carbon emitted from car exhausts for example. There is increasing evidence that the levels of these in the air are connected to morbidity and mortality. The smallest of these particles can penetrate deep into the lungs and may therefore contribute to lung diseases. As well as a strong association between levels of particulates and deaths from respiratory diseases, there is also a correlation with hospital admissions and reports of symptoms of asthma (Bown, 1994).

Acid Rain

In addition to having various effects on human health, pollutants may also be toxic to animals and plants in the environment and some of these effects can be demonstrated experimentally. One particular aspect of the environmental impact of pollutants currently of great concern is acid rain.

This term describes the wet precipitation of sulphuric and nitric acids and the dry deposition of sulphur dioxide, nitric acid and nitrogen oxides. It results from the burning of fossils fuels and certain industrial processes which produce sulphur dioxide and nitrogen oxides:

$$H_2O + SO_2 \xrightarrow{O_2;\ uv} H_2SO_4$$
$$\text{hydrocarbons}$$

$$NO_2 + H_2O \xrightarrow{H_2O;\ uv} HNO_3$$
$$\text{ozone}$$

These acids may be present in clouds and be removed during rain formation. This is known as washout. Alternatively they may be removed from the atmosphere by the falling rain. This is known as rain-out.

The effects of acid rain have been particularly noticeable in Scandinavia, partly as a result of the type of soil there. Sweden for example received about 472 000 tonnes of sulphur dioxide in 1980 but only produced 240 000 tonnes, some of which would be deposited in other neighbouring countries, so Sweden suffered a net gain of 230 000 tonnes, despite having reduced its own production from 300 000 tonnes in 1978. Acid rain is clearly a world-wide problem whereby the pollution is transported from one country to the next. Britain exports much of its pollution to Scandinavia and continental Europe (Figure 8.2) something which the Central Electricity Generating Board is now beginning to accept. Increased acidity has now been recognized in Britain itself, in Scotland and Snowdonia for example. The effects of acid rain depend on the type of deposition, the soil type and other factors. The buffering capacity of the soil is particularly important, but the thin soils found in parts of Scandinavia have poor buffering capacity and consequently the effects of the acidity are greater. The acidity in soil may also accumulate with time in some areas so that reducing the acid deposition will not have an immediate effect.

The sulphur and nitrogen oxides can cause rain, snow and mist to become acidic. Rain and snow mainly acidify the soil and ground water to a greater

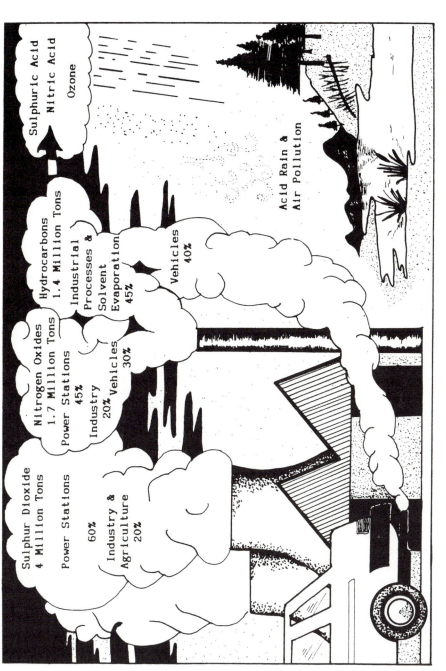

Figure 8.2. A graphic illustration of the problems of air pollution and of acid rain which occur in industrialized countries. The figures give an indication of the situation in Great Britain at one time.
Adapted from 'Why forests fear acid drops', *The Sunday Times*, 24 November 1985.

or lesser extent depending on the buffering capacity. The volume of rain or thaw water is also important for, if it is excessive, the water may overwhelm the natural buffers in the soil or saturate it. The water then runs straight into rivers and lakes with little contact with the bicarbonate and humus present in the soil which would buffer the acidity. Consequently, the rivers and lakes will become more acidic. Modern farming techniques, such as the use of ammonium sulphate fertilizers, may also exacerbate the increase in acidity. The actual acidity may cause certain organisms to die and will also upset the balance in the ecosystem. Water of low pH also leaches out metals such as cadmium and lead from the ground and causes aluminium salts to dissolve. These metals will damage plants if taken up by them and may also be toxic to animals. Cadmium is highly toxic to mammals, chronic exposure causing kidney damage and affecting bones in humans causing a brittle bone syndrome, which is known as Itai-Itai disease in Japan. Aluminium leached out of the soil and dissolved in acidic waters is believed to be one of the causes of the death of fish in Scandinavian lakes and rivers. One of the more vulnerable points is the reproductive cycle. How much damage wet deposition of acid causes to plants and especially trees is not yet clear. Dry deposition of sulphur dioxide, however, may damage leaves directly. There is serious damage to many types of trees in West Germany, and some estimate that 87 per cent of the firs are affected. This is now attributed to pollution. It may be due to a combination of factors and there is continuing discussion as to whether the major effect is acidification of the soil and release of toxic metals or direct damage to the leaves or needles. Clearly air pollution contains a number of different compounds, but it seems that ozone is the constituent which is more likely to be directly toxic to trees rather than sulphur dioxide. Acidic ground water will not only leach out toxic metals which will be taken up by the tree but it will also leach out essential nutrients and so the soil will become deficient in them.

Most scientists involved now agree that all of the constituents of pollution, from both power stations and cars, should be reduced as much as possible even though it is not yet clear which ones are the most important. However, some scientists and some Governments have argued that reducing sulphur dioxide, for example, may have little effect if the important determining factor is the level of ozone or hydrocarbons which catalyze the conversion of sulphur dioxide and nitrogen oxides to sulphuric acid and nitric acid respectively. It is possible, however, to remove some of the sulphur dioxide from the smoke derived from fossil fuels before, during and after burning. Similarly, the output of carbon monoxide, nitrogen oxides and hydrocarbons from car exhausts can be reduced with catalytic converters. These are already in use in some countries and in the USA emissions of carbon monoxide and hydrocarbons from new cars have fallen by 90 per cent and nitrogen oxides by 75 per cent between 1970 and 1983. Two of these pollutants, nitrogen oxides and hydrocarbons, are involved in the production of ozone in the atmosphere and nitrogen oxides also contribute to acid rain as already described. In the view of British scientists at Harwell, reducing hydrocarbons in car exhausts is the best way to reduce atmospheric ozone. It should be noted, however, that some ozone in the atmosphere is necessary and that if the atmospheric level drops too low then more ultraviolet light reaches the surface of the earth, possibly leading to an increase in skin cancer. The chlorofluorocarbons used as aerosol propellants are believed to be one cause of a *reduction* in atmospheric ozone.

Perhaps when the real extent and economic consequences of the damage due to these pollutants such as to buildings and metal structures as well as to trees and humans become known, governments will enact legislation to cause a major reduction in output pollutants from all sources.

Lead Pollution

Another major environmental pollutant is lead, known to be a poisonous compound for centuries. Its toxicity was certainly recognized by 300 BC as a case of lead poisoning was described by Hippocrates around that time. For centuries workers involved in lead mining and smelting have been occupationally exposed. Lead poisoning may even have contributed to the decline of the Roman Empire as high lead levels have been detected in Roman skeletons from that period. Lead pollution arises mainly from car exhausts but industrial processes, batteries, minerals and lead arsenate insecticide also contribute to lead in the environment. The use of cooking vessels with lead glaze or made of lead may have been another source in earlier times. Industrial poisoning became common in the Industrial Revolution, with a thousand cases a year in the UK alone at the end of the nineteenth century. However, a relatively recent study by the EEC in Glasgow showed that 10 per cent of babies had >0.3 μg ml^{-1} of lead in their blood indicating that there is still cause for concern. Lead is taken in from food, via the lungs and from water and although the amount found in food may be greater than that in air, the absorption is greater from the lungs than from the gut. Children are more susceptible than adults as they absorb greater amounts from the gastrointestinal tract.

It has been estimated that 98 per cent of the airborne lead in the UK is derived from leaded petrol and levels of lead in the air correlate with the amount of traffic. The lead in car exhausts is derived from tetraethyl lead, an anti-knock compound added to petrol which is converted to lead in the engine. Certain individuals, such as traffic policemen, may have higher blood lead levels than the average member of the urban population because they have greater exposure to car exhausts. Cigarette smoke is also a source of inhaled lead.

At the beginning of the twentieth century large-scale poisoning of children with lead became known, especially of those living in poor housing in slum areas of the USA. The source of this lead was mainly from paint containing relatively large amounts of lead. The paint was taken in by children through contamination of food or fingers or perhaps by experimental tasting of flakes of paint. In children, the most serious effect of lead poisoning is encephalopathy with mental retardation, and seizures and cerebral palsy may be lifelong effects. The nervous system is a clear target for lead and is particularly susceptible in young children. A cause for concern is whether even a single episode of poisoning is sufficient to cause permanent damage in children.

After absorption, lead enters the blood where 97 per cent is taken up by the red blood cell. The half-life of lead in the red blood cell is 2–3 weeks. Some redistribution of the lead to liver and kidney occurs and then excretion into the bile or deposition in bone takes place. In bone the lead eventually becomes incorporated into the hydroxyapatite crystal. Due to this deposition in bone and teeth it is possible to estimate past exposure to lead by X-ray analysis. It is also possible to detect lead poisoning and exposure from urine and blood analysis as the amount in blood represents the current exposure.

The 'normal' blood levels in the USA have been reported as between $0.15–0.7 \mu g \ ml^{-1}$ with an average at $0.3 \mu g \ ml^{-1}$. The threshold for toxicity is $0.8 \mu g \ ml^{-1}$, and encephalopathy occurs at $1–2 \mu g \ ml^{-1}$. However, biochemical effects can be seen at lower levels: lead interferes with haem and porphyrin synthesis and its effects on the enzymes of this pathway can be demonstrated (Figure 8.3); myoglobin synthesis and cytochrome P-450 may also be affected. The results of the effects on porphyrin synthesis are a reduction in haemoglobin level, the appearance of coproporphyrin and aminolaevulinic acid (ALA) in the urine. Free erythrocyte protoporphyrin is increased and aminolaevulinic acid dehydrase (ALAD) is inhibited. Inhibition of ALAD is the most sensitive measure of exposure and in human subjects there is a correlation between blood lead and the degree of inhibition of the enzyme. At blood levels of $0.4 \mu g \ ml^{-1}$ ALAD is inhibited to the extent of 50 per cent. At levels of $0.6–0.8 \mu g \ ml^{-1}$ there is a greater effect and mild symptoms; at levels of $0.8–1.0 \mu g \ ml^{-1}$ there are more definite clinical signs;

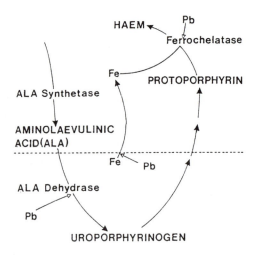

Figure 8.3. The synthesis of haem in the mammalian erythrocyte. The points at which lead (Pb) interferes with this synthetic pathway are shown.

at levels of $1-2\ \mu g\ ml^{-1}$ encephalopathy occurs. The symptoms are non-specific colic and abdominal pain, lassitude and constipation. Anaemia occurs later and CNS effects occur after prolonged exposure. The blood lead level rises and ALAD falls within a few days of exposure. The ALA and coproporphyrin in urine increase after two weeks.

Lead interferes at several steps in haem synthesis: with the enzymes ferrochelatase, aminolaevulinate synthetase (ALAS) and aminolaevulinate dehydrase (ALAD), and with the uptake of iron into the mitochondrion. Increased excretion of ALA in the urine is one marker for lead exposure. In 1970 10 per cent of all children in New York and Chicago had blood levels of $0.6\ \mu g\ ml^{-1}$. Many of these children lived in good housing. As with carbon monoxide exposure anaemic individuals who have a low haemoglobin level and reduced red blood cell count may be more at risk as their lead carrying capacity is lower and the amount of haemoglobin is already low. Anaemia may result from lead exposure partly as a result of inhibition of haemoglobin synthesis and partly by causing the destruction of red blood cells.

Measurement of the inhibition of ALAD is too sensitive a measure of lead exposure, whereas the presence of haemoglobin and copropophyrin in urine occurs after severe damage. The detection of ALA in urine is the most useful method for determination of lead poisoning.

As well as affecting the CNS and haem synthesis, in children lead also causes skeletal changes following chronic exposure. Bands at the growing ends of long bones can be detected and bone shape may also be affected. Chronic exposure may also be detected by a lead line on the gums. Acute exposure to lead may also cause kidney damage, while chronic exposure may lead to interstitial nephritis. This may be the cause of the nephritis associated with drinking moonshine whisky as the stills used sometimes contained lead piping or lead solder.

Whether lead in the atmosphere in cities poses a real threat to the mental health of children is currently disputed. Barltrop does not believe that the data shows there is a clear relationship between the body lead burden and IQ decreases in children but it may be difficult to prove such a relationship. In the UK there have been three reports on this: by the DHSS, by a Royal Commission and by the Medical Research Council; all have concluded that many of the studies on this aspect of lead poisoning were inadequate. Studies are under way to look at blood lead levels of $0.4-0.8\ \mu g\ ml^{-1}$ in relation to the function of the central and peripheral nervous system. It has been suggested that subclinical disease of the central and peripheral nervous system and kidney may follow long-term exposure at levels to which the general population are exposed in the urban environment. This is very difficult, however, if not impossible to prove in the human population.

So far we have been considering inorganic lead, yet organic lead is probably more toxic as it is lipid-soluble and therefore well absorbed. For example, triethyl lead which results from combustion of petrol containing tetraethyl lead, is readily taken up through skin and into the brain and will cause encephalopathy. This has been the cause of toxic effects in workers exposed in industry where the tetraethyl lead is manufactured. The effects occur rapidly and the symptoms are delusions, hallucinations and ataxia.

How much of a hazard the levels of lead in our air, food and water pose to the health of children and adults is currently unclear. However, it is probable that we could remove much of that pollution and the hazard by removing lead from petrol without any major effect on petrol prices or car performance. Lead is known from both animal and human studies to be highly toxic and the levels to which many of us are exposed can be shown to have effects on biochemical pathways. It is surely only prudent to reduce the exposure to this toxic metal as much as possible by reducing its use and release into the environment.

Water Pollution

Water in rivers, lakes and the sea may be polluted directly by the discharge of effluent from factories and industrial processes, and of domestic waste. Water may become polluted also by substances on the land such as pesticides and fertilizers applied to crops and washed by rain into rivers and lakes and eventually into the sea. The rain can also directly accumulate substances from the atmosphere. Industrial companies may dump toxic waste into underground storage tanks and leakage of these has been known to lead to contamination of the water table. The domestic water supply in such areas then becomes contaminated.

Some water pollutants, such as fertilizers from agricultural run-off, sewage and organic waste products from the food industry lead to overgrowth of algae and other aquatic plants which eventually choke the local environment and use up the available nutrients. The algae then die, and decay with the help of aerobic bacteria which use up the oxygen in the water. This is followed by the appearance of anaerobic bacteria which continue to feed from the decaying plant matter at the bottom of the lake or river. These bacteria produce toxic compounds which, along with the lack of oxygen, cause the water to become stagnant and so other aquatic organisms such as fish die. This process is known as eutrophication.

Humans, other animals and plants may become exposed to toxic pollutants in water either by drinking that water, living in it or eating other organisms which have become contaminated by it. Although in Western nations drinking water is normally highly purified, this may not be the case in less developed countries. However some toxic substances, such as heavy metals, are not necessarily removed by the normal water-treatment procedures.

Water pollutants may affect organisms within the environment in different ways. High concentrations of a toxic compound may kill most or all of the organisms within a particular area where the concentration is sufficiently high. However, this area may become repopulated in time from another area. A more insidious pollutant may damage the reproductive cycle of certain organisms in some way. Fish eggs are very susceptible to toxic compounds at low levels for example and this may lead to a decline in the fish population.

Another way in which a pollutant can interact with the environment is by entering food chains (see below), without causing damage to the lower organisms in the chain, but possibly killing the predators at the top of the chain or interfering with their reproductive cycle. Persistent compounds such as methyl mercury and DDT enter food chains and act in this way.

The pollutant may not however remain the same once it is in the environment as it may be altered by chemical or biochemical processes. Consequently, two important aspects of environmental pollution are the involvement of food chains and the alteration of the compound by the environment itself.

Food Chains

For a terrestrial animal the most likely route of exposure to a toxic compound such as a pollutant is via its food. The food chain is one method by which animals and man become exposed to persistent pollutants. Substances may however be persistent in one environment or species but not in another, depending on the particular characteristics of the system. The food chain can involve water-borne pollutants and also soil and airborne pollutants. There are two main types of food chain; grazing and detritivore. A grazing food chain is a sequence in which one organism, such as a plant, is eaten by another such as a herbivore which is in turn eaten by a carnivore and so on (Table 7.3). A detritivore food chain involves the decay of organisms after death. The organisms involved tend to be small and there is no increase in size between the lower and higher trophic levels. Both types of food chain can be involved in environmental toxicology as can other types of feeding relationships. The overall system may be termed a food web.

The amounts of a pollutant in species at each trophic level (Table 7.3) may be measured and compared to give a concentration factor. However, these must be interpreted with caution. For example, the mode of sampling a population may have inherent bias. Ideally sampling should be random, but it may not always be so. If animal carcasses are sampled the levels of a particular pollutant may vary widely depending on the cause of death. Indeed the concentration of pollutant in live animals may be at least as important as the concentration in those dying of unknown cause. This is because the pollutant may have subtle population effects, such as on breeding behaviour or the production of eggs, which will affect the whole population. Another important point is that the mere presence of a chemical in the environment does not necessarily mean there has been significant pollution and similarly the presence of a chemical in an organism does not necessarily mean that it is causing toxic effects. Our ability to measure toxic compounds at minute levels should not blind us to the necessity for a reasonable assessment and interpretation of those data. Unlike controlled laboratory experiments, environmental exposure may often be intermittent and pollutants do not always reach a steady state but can fluctuate wildly. As already mentioned, persistence of a chemical can vary between species or ecosystems. For example, it has been reported that small mammals may have a low level of organochlorine insecticides whilst birds feeding on them may have very high and possibly lethal levels. This may be due to differences in the metabolism of the pollutant by the two species.

Thus, the mammal might eliminate the substance relatively rapidly whereas the bird may not and so it will accumulate. Again sampling can be an important factor in studying this problem as predators may take prey from a wide area in which there are great variations in exposure. It is clear that environmental toxicology deals with complex systems in which prediction is sometimes very difficult.

Although the effects of pollutants on individual human beings may be perceived by man as the most important, ecologically and biologically an effect on the population may be more important. Consequently, a pollutant which reduces or stops reproduction of the species at some stage is more important than a pollutant which is more acutely toxic but only causes the death of the older, more susceptible members of that species. The latter would be more obviously distressing but would have less effect on the population if the victims were past significant reproductive capacity. The toxic compound would be just one more cause of death. Indeed not all individuals in a population reproduce and so there may be less effect than might be expected for a toxic pollutant which leads to the death of only some members of that population.

An example which illustrates this effect on the reproductive cycle and the problems of persistent pesticides in food chains is the effect of organochlorine insecticides on eggshells in predatory birds, as mentioned in Chapter 7. The predatory bird is at the top of a food chain and hence may have the highest concentration of pollutant. The peregrine falcon population in Britain declined precipitately between 1955 and 1962. At the same time the frequency of egg breakage increased because of a decrease in eggshell thickness. There is a linear relationship between eggshell strength and the thickness index. Peregrine falcon eggs studied during the period 1970–1974 had a lower thickness index and strength than those studied between 1850 and 1942. DDE, a metabolite of DDT is believed to be one cause of this decreased thickness. Direct toxicity of dieldrin to falcons has been suggested as another cause of the decline in population. Areas such as the north of Scotland had a higher eggshell thickness index and lower levels of DDE than eggs from more southern areas of the UK. Similarly data from the USA for kestrels showed a correlation between eggshell thickness and DDE concentration (Figure 7.2).

Pollutants which contaminate water may either dissolve in it if they are ionized/water-soluble substances or are miscible. Alternatively if they are hydrophobic they may form a suspension or aggregate and remain undispersed in the same manner as the familiar oil slick. Although water-soluble substances may reach a sufficient concentration to be toxic to aquatic organisms and to man, unless they are in an enclosed system they will tend to disperse eventually. Such compounds are not likely to accumulate in organisms. Hydrophobic substances however behave differently. Substances which are not polar and are soluble in lipid rather than water are well absorbed by living organisms especially by aquatic organisms which pass water over gills to extract oxygen and to filter water in search of food. Consequently, small organisms such as *Daphnia* and zooplankton become contaminated with lipophilic pollutants such as DDT. These small organisms are then eaten by other, larger organisms such as small fish and the contaminant enters the fatty tissue of this larger organism. However, if the small organisms are ingested in large numbers and the compound is not readily excreted, the concentration of the substance in the larger organism increases. This process is repeated with ever larger and larger organisms until the ultimate predator, at the top of the food chain may accumulate sufficient of the substance to suffer toxic effects (Table 7.3; Figure 8.4). Food chains may occur in aquatic environments with water pollutants, or in terrestrial organisms with airborne, soil, water or food borne pollutants, or a combination of these. The important aspect of any food chain, therefore, is the scope for biomagnification of the substance as it moves up through the chain. Furthermore the compound may be non-toxic at the low levels encountered by the organisms at the bottom of the chain which therefore survive and contaminate the predators further up the chain.

The most important characteristics of a substance which enters a food chain are its lipid solubility and its metabolic stability in biological systems. These determine the extent to which the compound is taken up by the organism and its ability to localize in fat tissue and remain there until the organism is ingested by a predator. Hydrophilic compounds, which are polar and ionized may be taken up by organisms but will tend to be readily excreted. Lipophilic pollutants which are absorbed and then rapidly metabolized to polar metabolites similarly tend to be readily excreted and hence will not persist in the organism or be transferred to the predator.

This is another example of the importance of physico-chemical characteristics in toxicology.

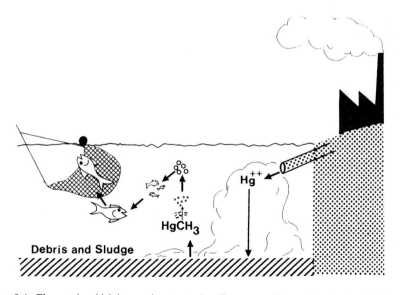

Figure 8.4. The way in which inorganic mercury in effluent was taken up into the food chain and lead to the poisoning of several hundred local inhabitants in Minamata Bay in Japan. The inorganic mercury was methylated by micro-organisms in the anaerobic sludge lying at the bottom of the bay and so became more soluble in fatty tissue and was easily taken up into living organisms.

Although some environmental pollutants are not lipophilic initially they may be metabolized by micro-organisms, plants or higher animals to lipophilic metabolites which are more persistent. DDT is an example of this; its metabolite DDE is more lipophilic and much more persistent (Figure 7.1 and Table 7.2). Another is inorganic mercury (see below).

We will now consider an example of an environmental pollutant where such factors are involved.

Mercury and Methylmercury

Mercury is 'the hottest, the coldest, a true healer, a wicked murderer, a precious medicine, and a deadly poison, a friend that can flatter and lie.' (Woodall, J. (1639) *The Surgeon' Mate or Military & Domestic Surgery*. London, p. 256, quoted from *Cassarett and Doull's Toxicology*.)

Like lead, mercury is a highly toxic metal the toxic properties of which have been known about for centuries. The phrase 'Mad as a Hatter' has its origins in the effects on exposed workers of the mercury salts used to cure felt for hats. Mercury and its salts have been used in many ways for centuries. In the Middle Ages it was used to treat syphilis.

Mercury exists in three chemical forms: elemental, inorganic and organic. All three forms are toxic in different ways. Elemental mercury (Hg^0), often used in scientific instruments, is absorbed as the vapour and is highly toxic. Mercury readily vaporizes even at room temperature and exposure to it can lead to damage to the central nervous system. Inorganic mercury (Hg^+ and Hg^{2+}), in mercury salts, is not readily absorbed but when it does gain access to the body, it causes mainly kidney damage. Organic mercury compounds ($R\text{-}Hg^+$) are readily absorbed by living organisms and, therefore, are more hazardous than inorganic mercury. As with elemental mercury, the target is the brain and nervous system.

The different forms of mercury may act by basically similar mechanisms of action involving the reaction of the metal or its ions with sulphydryl groups. These sulphydryl groups may be part of a protein, such as an enzyme, and hence mercury is a potent inhibitor of enzymes in which the SH group is important. The differences in the toxicity of the three forms of mercury are due to differences in distribution. Elemental mercury is readily taken up from the lungs and is oxidized in red blood cells to Hg^{2+}. Hg^0 is also readily taken up into the brain and the foetus and is also metabolized to Hg^{2+} in these tissues. The mercury is then trapped in these sites by virtue of being ionized. Consequently elemental mercury causes mainly neurological damage. Inorganic mercury cannot cross the blood-brain barrier, but reaches the kidney and it is this organ particularly that is damaged. Organic mercury is sufficiently lipid-soluble to distribute to the central nervous system where it also is oxidized to Hg^{2+}, and causes mainly neurological damage. So, although all three forms of mercury are probably toxic as a result of binding to sulphydryl groups in proteins, the differences in distribution lead to differences in the type of toxicity. This is another illustration of the importance of distribution in the toxicity of foreign compounds.

Exposure to mercury used to be mainly an occupational hazard rather than an environmental one, but more recently mercury has also become an environmental pollutant. This has occurred through the use of organomercury fungicides and through the industrial use of mercury in the manufacture of plastics, paper and batteries with the resultant discharge of the contaminated effluents into lakes and rivers. High levels have been detected, as in water near a battery plant in Michigan, where levels of 1000 ppm were found when the permissible level was 5 ppb. Mercury has also been detected in air, presumably arising from industrial processes.

Dumping of the inorganic form of the metal used to be tolerated because it was thought that this form was relatively innocuous and easily dispersed.

The use of mercury-containing fungicides has led to water contamination via run-off from fields. Other sources of environmental mercury are wood pulp plants and chloroalkali plants. These and possibly other sources were presumably responsible for the contamination of freshwater fish by high levels of mercury detected by Swedish scientists. As with other lipid-soluble substances in the environment, bioconcentration in the food chain also occurs.

Mercury dumping is now controlled and organomercury fungicides are being phased out.

A tragic and now infamous event, which occurred in Japan in the 1950s, highlighted the dangers of inorganic mercury as a water pollutant. In 1956 a new factory on the shores of Minamata Bay in Japan began producing vinyl chloride and acetaldehyde. Mercuric chloride was used as a catalyst, and after use was discharged into the bay with the rest of the effluent from the factory. Within a year a new illness had appeared among the local fishermen and their families which became known as Minamata Disease. Their pet cats also suffered similar symptoms. It was eventually recognized that the disease was due to contaminated seafood and mercury was suspected in 1959. Methylmercury was detected in seafood in 1960 and in sediments derived from the factory in 1961. The methylmercury was being taken up by the seafood which was eaten by the local population. A food chain was involved with the organic mercury being concentrated by the aquatic organisms because, unlike inorganic mercury it is lipid-soluble. It became apparent that the inorganic mercury that discharged into rivers, lakes or the sea was not inert but could be biomethylated to methylmercury by micro-organisms (Figure 8.4). This occurred especially under anaerobic conditions, such as in the effluent sludge which collected at the bottom of Minamata Bay. This highlighted the fact that inorganic mercury dumped into rivers and lakes is by no means innocuous and is not necessarily dispersed.

The contamination at Minamata led to 700 cases of poisoning and over 70 deaths. Diversion of effluent by the factory eliminated the disease. Mass poisonings have also occurred in various parts of the world as a result of the use of organomercury compounds as fungicides to treat seed grain. The treated grain should not be used as food but if it is used to feed livestock, the meat becomes contaminated. One such large-scale poisoning incident occurred in Iraq in 1971–1972 when alkylmercury fungicides were used to treat cereal grain. This involved 6000 people and resulted in 500 deaths.

In another incident in 1969, a New Mexico family fed treated grain to pigs, and then ate the pigs. Three of the ten children exposed experienced behavioural abnormalities and other neurological disorders. A child exposed *in utero* was born with brain damage and the urinary level of mercury was found to be 15 times that of the mother.

The symptoms of methylmercury poisoning reflect the entry of the compound into the central nervous system, beginning with memory loss, paresthesias, ataxia, narrowing of the visual field, and progressing to loss of muscle co-ordination and emotional instability and eventually cerebral palsy. The latter was the most distressing effect seen at Minamata. Children and new born infants seemed to be most severely affected and those exposed *in utero* were born with severe cerebral palsy even when the mothers were symptom-free, a classic characteristic of a teratogen. Methylmercury is able to cross the placenta and may consequently concentrate in the fat tissue and brain of the embryo and foetus. In addition, foetal red blood cells concentrate methyl-mercury 30 per cent more than the adult red blood cells. The damage caused by methylmercury is permanent.

The methylmercury that enters the brain is demethylated and the inorganic mercury released can then bind to the sulphydryl groups of enzymes and inactivate them. Methylmercury has a long half-life in the body, approximately 70 days. It is localized particularly in the liver and brain, with 10–20 per cent of the body burden of mercury in the brain. It is possible to calculate from this and the known toxic concentration that the allowable daily intake with a safety factor of 10 would be 0.1 mg day^{-1} This would correspond

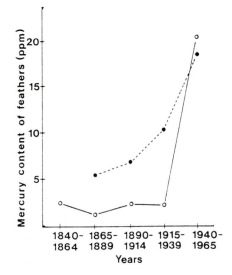

Figure 8.5. The increase in mercury levels detected in two species of birds, Crested Grebe (●) and Goshawk (○), over a 100-year period. The mercury content was determined in feathers from museum specimens of Swedish birds.
Data from Wallace *et al.* (1971) Mercury in the Environment: The Human Element, ORNL-NSF Environmental Program Oak Ridge National Laboratory, Figure 4.

to eating 200 g of fish with a mercury level of 0.5 ppm, but fish in Lake Michigan and in the sea off the coast of Sweden has been found to contain as much as ten times more mercury than this in some cases.

Like humans, birds and other animals may ingest mercury. For example, studies of the crested Grebe show that tissue mercury levels have been steadily increasing since about 1870 (Figure 8.5).

Substances, such as pesticides and other chemicals, which may contaminate the environment have to be tested for toxicity in a variety of species including fish, Daphnia, honey bees and earthworms. Also, ecotoxicity testing requires determination of the biochemical and chemical oxygen demand, abbreviated BOD and COD respectively. The BOD indicates the ability of micro-organisms to metabolize an organic substance. The COD is the amount of oxygen required to oxidize the substance chemically. The ratio of the COD and BOD is an indication of the biodegradability of the substance. There are a number of other tests which will give an indication of the persistence of the compound in the environment such as determination of abiotic degradation. Details of these can be found in the documents issued by such governmental organizations as the Environmental Protection Agency (EPA) in the USA and the Health and Safety Executive (HSE) in Britain.

Questions

1. Briefly describe with examples the toxicological importance of the following

    (a) acid rain;
    (b) food chains;
    (c) biomagnification.

2. Describe the major causes, sources and consequences for human health of air pollution.

3. Discuss the human toxicology of either (a) lead or (b) mercury in relation to environmental exposure.

Bibliography

Amdur, M. O. (1991) Air pollutants, in *Cassarett and Doull's Toxicology*, Amdur, M. O., Doull, J. and Klaassen, C. (Eds), 4th edition, New York: Pergamon Press.

Barltrop, D. (1985) Lead and Brain Damage, *Human Toxicology*, **4**: 121.

Bown, W. (1994) Dying from too much dust, *New Scientists*, **141** (1916), 12–13.

Francis, B. M. (1994) *Toxic Substances in the Environment. An Overview of Environmental Toxicology*. New York: John Wiley.

Guthrie, F. E. and Perry, J. J. (Eds) (1980) *Introduction to Environmental Toxicology*, New York: Elsevier.

Maynard, R. L. and Waller, R. E. (1993) Air pollution, in Ballantyne, B., Marrs, T. and Turner, P. (Eds), *General and Applied Toxicology*, Basingstoke, UK: Macmillan.

Menzer, R. E. (1991) Water and soil pollutants, in *Cassarett and Doull's Toxicology*, Amdur, M. O., Doull, J. and Klaassen, C. (Eds), 4th edition, New York: Pergamon Press.

Moriarty, F. (1988) *Ecotoxicology: The Study of Pollutants in Ecosystems*, 2nd edition, London: Academic Press.

Owens, R. V. and Owens, R. (1983) *Acidification of the Environment Including Acid Raid*, Powys: Pyramid.

Peakall, D. B. (1994) Biomarkers: the way forward in environmental assessment, *Toxicology and Ecotoxicology News*, **1**, 55–60.

Pearce, F. (1987) Acid rain, *New Scientist*, 5 November, 1–4.

Rand, G. M. and Petrocelli, S. R. (1985) *Fundamentals of Aquatic Toxicology*, Washington, DC: Hemisphere.

Zakrewski, S. F. (1991) *Principles of Environmental Toxicology*, Washington, DC: American Chemical Society.

Chapter 9

Natural Products

Although many of the toxic chemicals in the environment that worry the general public are man-made, there are also many hundreds of natural poisons of animal, plant, fungal and microbial origin. Indeed, the most toxic substances known to man are natural poisons such as botulinum toxin (Table 1.1) and it is certainly not reasonable to imply, as do some of the advertisements for health foods and herbal medicines, that natural substances are intrinsically harmless and safe. For example, allergies to natural constituents of food are known to occur just as they do to synthetic additives. Some of these natural, toxic substances have been known about for centuries and have been used for murder or suicide, or even sometimes misguided medical treatment (see Chapter 1).

Natural substances also still occasionally feature in accidental poisoning cases although this is relatively rare compared with poisoning by drug overdose. Natural toxins are of diverse structure and mode of action, and there are far too many categories to consider each individually in this book. Consequently we will simply examine a few interesting and important examples of toxic substances derived from plants, animals, fungi and micro-organisms.

Plant Toxins

There are many well known plant toxins ranging from the irritant formic acid found in nettles (and ants) to more poisonous compounds such as atropine in deadly nightshade berries (*Atropa belladonna*), cytisine in laburnam and coniine in hemlock. Let us consider a few less well-known plant toxins which have been studied recently.

Pyrrolizidine Alkaloids

There is a group of these alkaloids which are produced by plants of the *Senecio, Heliotropium* and *Crotolaria* species, many of which occur as weeds throughout the world. The plants have on occasion contaminated cereal crops and human consumption of flour made from them led to poisoning. This has occurred in various parts of the world, especially where agricultural conditions are poor and the indigenous population may be forced to use the contaminated crops. For example, in South Africa during the 1930s poor whites suffered the toxic effects of these alkaloids because their staple diet was wheat which became contaminated, whereas their Bantu neighbours, who ate maize which was not contaminated, were not affected. More recently, poisonings have occurred in Tashkent, Central India and Northern Afghanistan. In one incident where 1600 poisoning cases were reported, the threshed wheat was found to be contaminated with *Heliotropium popovii* seeds giving an alkaloid concentration of at least 0.5 per cent. In the West Indies especially, these plants may also be used in traditional medicine to make herbal teas.

These alkaloids are interesting because after acute exposure, such as after the ingestion of herbal teas, they cause a particular form of liver disease known as veno-occlusive disease. The effect of chronic exposure to low doses is liver cirrhosis which can be seen in some members of the West Indian population, estimated to account for one third of the cirrhosis seen at autopsy in Jamaica. The constituent alkaloids, such as monocrotaline which has been extensively studied, (Figure 9.1), undergo metabolic activation to a reactive metabolite which damages the cells lining the liver sinusoids as well as the hepatocytes, leading to haemorrhagic necrosis and finally to the veno-occlusive disease. This blockage of the blood vessels in the liver eventually gives rise to alteration of the vasculature such that the liver blood supply is diverted and new blood vessels grow.

Animals may also be exposed and suffer the toxic effects. Where there is abundant vegetation for grazing, animals will ignore plants such as ragwort (*Senecio jacoboea*) which contain the alkaloids but in some countries, such as Australia, widespread losses of horses, cattle and sheep have occurred from heliotropium poisoning. This may also be another route of human exposure as the alkaloids can be detected in the milk of cows grazing on such plants.

Pennyroyal Oil

The Pennyroyal plant and the oil prepared from it have been used to induce abortions in the USA where it is possible to buy the oil 'over the counter'. The plant may be used to make a tea or the oil may be taken directly. Both may cause toxic effects, especially liver damage as well as inducing abortion. The

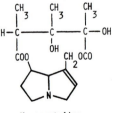

Monocrotaline

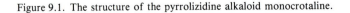

Figure 9.1. The structure of the pyrrolizidine alkaloid monocrotaline.

oil contains a number of terpenoid compounds and metabolic activation is believed to be required for the toxicity.

Ricin

Ricin is a highly toxic plant product found in the seeds of the castor oil plant. It achieved some notoriety when it was claimed that it had been used by the Bulgarian secret police to kill the Bulgarian journalist Georgi Markov in London in 1978. Although no trace of any poison was found in the victim's body clearly an extremely potent poison had been used and the symptoms were consistent with those of ricin poisoning. A tiny metal pellet was recovered from a wound on the victim's leg, seemingly inflicted accidentally by an umbrella. The pellet almost certainly was a reservoir for a toxic substance, but it could only contain a few nanograms of the substance.

Ricin is a small protein consisting of two polypeptides, a short A chain and a longer B chain. The A and B chains are linked via a disulphide bridge. The B chain attaches the ricin molecule to the outside of the mammalian cell by binding to the galactose part of a glycoprotein. The cell membrane invaginates and the ricin is taken into the cell inside a vacuole. The ricin molecule is released from the glycoprotein and the A and B chains then break at the disulphide bridge. The B chain makes a channel through the vacuole cell wall, allowing the A chain to enter the cytoplasm and reach the ribosomes where it blocks protein synthesis and kills the cell. One molecule of ricin is sufficient to kill one cell.

Bracken

The bracken fern contains a substance, ptaquiloside, which degrades into a compound which is carcinogenic. In Japan, the shoots of the bracken fern are eaten and this may explain the high incidence of throat cancer among the Japanese. Animals which eat the fern as fodder suffer from bladder and intestinal cancer. The breakdown product of ptaquiloside reacts with DNA, specifically the base adenine, and this is lost with the result that the DNA chain breaks.

Fluoroacetate

For a description of the toxicity of this naturally occuring plant toxin see Chapter 7.

There are many more well-known substances derived from plants such as the drugs heroin, morphine, cannabis, nicotine and digitalis.

Animal Toxins

As with plant toxins, animal toxins comprise a diverse range of structures and modes of action (Figure 9.2). A simple and well-known example is formic acid

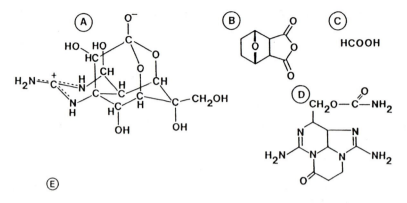

Figure 9.2. The structures of various animal toxins. A: tetrodotoxin; B: cantharidin; C: formic acid; D: saxitoxin; E: Amino acid sequence from honey bee venom phospholipase A.

which is found in ants (the name is derived from the Latin word, *formica*, for an ant). Other examples are tetrodotoxin found in the Puffer Fish and saxitoxin found in shellfish and fish which have consumed certan dinoflagellates. Animal toxins are often mixtures of complex proteins. Most of us suffer from animal toxins at some time in our lives even if it is only a wasp or bee sting. However, in some countries death and illness due to animal poisons represents an important proportion of poisoning cases and a significant cause of illness and death.

Snake venoms

Snake bites are one of the most common forms of poisoning by natural toxins worldwide. Many snake venoms are similar in their mode of action and constituents, being mixtures of proteins or polypeptides. The proteins may be enzymes, especially hydrolytic enzymes. Some of the more important are proteinases, phospholipases, ribonucleases, deoxyribonucleases, phospho-monoesterases and phosphodiesterases, and ATPases. The toxicity of some snake venoms is shown in Table. 9.1. The venoms may be mixtures and consequently cause a variety of effects. For example, the presence of foreign proteins may cause an anaphylactic reaction, although this is rare, and such allergic reactions may cause death in minutes. The enzyme components can digest various tissue constituents either at the site of action, causing local necrosis, or elsewhere causing systemic effects. For example, the bite of the diamondback rattlesnake, the most poisonous snake in the USA produces a very painful swelling within minutes. Nausea, vomiting and diarrhoea may occur and cardiac effects, such as a fall in systemic arterial blood pressure and a weak, rapid pulse, may be seen. The central nervous system can be affected, leading to respiratory paralysis. Haemolytic anaemia and haemoglobinuria sometimes occur, and there may be thrombosis and haemorrhage. Vascular permeability and nerve conduction can change, and cerebral anoxia, pulmonary oedema and heart failure also develop. The phospholipases found in snake venom sometimes cause intravascular haemolysis by direct action on the red cell membrane.

Most snake venoms contain a phosphodiesterase which attacks polynucleotides.

Tetrodotoxin

This toxin is found in the Puffer Fish and also in the Californian newt and has been studied extensively. The fish is eaten as a delicacy in Japan and provided it is properly prepared is edible and safe. However, fatalities have occurred which resulted from incorrect preparation of the fish and about 60 per cent of poisoning cases are fatal. The tetrodotoxin and another toxin ichthyocrinotoxin are found in the roe, liver and skin of the fish. Tetrodotoxin is a very potent nerve poison, lethal at doses of around 10 μg kg^{-1} body weight. Initial effects are a tingling in the mouth followed within 10–45 minutes by muscular inco-ordination, salivation, skin numbness, vomiting, diarrhoea and convulsions. Death results from skeletal muscle paralysis. Sensory as well as motor nerves are affected and it is believed that tetrodotoxin selectively blocks

Table 9.1. Comparative toxicity of snake venoms.

Snake venom	Yield (g)	LD$_{50}$ i.v. mg/kg
Copperhead	40–72	10.92
African puff adder	130–200	3.68
Mojave rattler	50–90	0.21
Russell's viper	130–250	0.08
Sea snake	7–20	0.01

Source: F. W. Oehme, J. F. Brown and M. E. Fowler (1980), Toxins of animal origin, in *Cassarett and Doull's Toxicology*, J. Doull, C. D. Klaassen and M. O. Amdur (Eds), 2nd edition, New York: Macmillan.

the sodium channels along the axon, preventing the inward action potential current.

Fungal Toxins

Many fungi produce toxins of a variety of chemical types and these can cause acute or chronic poisoning. Poisonous mushrooms may be confused with the edible varieties and hence accidental acute poisoning may occur. Poisoning may also occur through the intentional eating of fungi believed to contain psychoactive substances. Several fungal toxins have been fully identified and characterized. The toxic effects vary from relatively mild gastrointestinal disturbances to severe organ damage. Some, such as the psychoactive consti-tuents mescaline and psilocin, affect the central nervous system. Certain fungal products, such as the aflatoxins which are discussed in Chapter 6, are potent carcinogens.

Death Cap Mushroom

The Death Cap mushroom, *Amanita phalloides* is probably the most poisonous mushroom in Britain. It is occasionally eaten by mistake, but poisoning with this mushroom is rare in the UK. The mushroom contains a number of toxins: the phallotoxins, including phalloidin, phalloin and phallo-lysin, and the amatoxins (α, β and γ amanitin). The phallotoxins cause violent gastroenteritis which occurs rapidly (4–8 hours) after the mushroom is eaten.

The amatoxins have a delayed toxic effect, with the liver and kidney as target organs; liver necrosis and destruction of renal tubular cells may result. Both the phallotoxins and the amanitins are strongly bound to plasma proteins yet are toxic in this form. Consequently, treatment involves displacement from the proteins by a drug such as a sulphonamide or benzylpenicillin which will reduce toxicity. This is probably due to increased excretion of the unbound form as protein binding of foreign compounds slows excretion (see Chapter 2).

After the mushroom is eaten sometimes there may not be any symptoms for up to a day then vomiting and diarrhoea occur possibly followed by jaundice, hypoglycaemia, acidosis and other effects on blood chemistry. In severe cases hepatic failure can result.

Aflatoxins

These fungal toxins have already been discussed under food contaminants (Chapter 6). Aflatoxin B1 causes liver damage after high doses but in humans chronic exposure to lower doses via the diet is a more likely occurrence which can cause liver tumours. The toxin is most likely to occur in food infected with the mould *Aspergillus flavus* or prepared from infected food or ingredients.

Microbial Toxins

There are many toxins produced by bacteria. As with other natural toxins, they are of a variety of chemical types and consequently they cause a variety of different toxic effects, ranging from gastrointestinal effects to severe and fatal effects on the nervous system. We will consider just one well known toxic syndrome, botulism.

Botulism and Botulinum Toxin

The toxic bacterial product botulinum toxin is produced by the bacterium *Clostridium botulinum*. The syndrome this causes is known as botulism and results from oral ingestion of the toxin. The bacteria thrive under anaerobic conditions and produce a mixture of six heat-labile toxins. Consequently, botulism is often produced by a bacterial infection of home- canned or bottled non-acid foodstuffs which have become infected during preparation, have been inadequately preserved and not refrigerated, and have not been adequately heated prior to eating. The toxin itself is destroyed by heating although the spores of the bacterium are quite heat-resistant.

This toxin is one of the most potent known to man, with an LD_{50} of around 0.01 $\mu g\ kg^{-1}$ and so less than a microgram would be lethal for a human. It acts on the nerve terminal, binding irreversibly to it and preventing the release of acetylcholine. The result of this is that the muscle behaves as if it was denervated and the victim suffers paralysis and fatal cessation of breathing if severe. Although botulism may prove fatal fortunately such poisoning is relatively uncommon.

Question

1. Write short notes related to the toxicology of three of the following:

    (a) pyrrolizidine alkaloids;
    (b) ricin;
    (c) snake venoms;
    (d) tetrodotoxin;
    (e) *Amanita phalloides*.

Bibliography

Emsley, J. (1994) How bracken's deadly chemical breaks the back of DNA, *New Scientist*, **142** (1921), 16.

Habermeyl, G. G. (1981) *Venomous Animals and Their Toxins*, Berlin: Springer Verlag.

Harris, J. B. (Ed.) (1986) *Natural Toxins, Animal, Plant and Microbial*, Oxford: Oxford University Press.

HMSO (1987) Mycotoxins, Food Surveillance Paper no. 18, London: HMSO.

Lampe, K. F. (1991) Toxic effects of plant toxins, in *Cassarett and Doull's Toxicology*, Amdur, M. O., Doull, J. and Klaassen, C. (Eds), 4th edition, New York: Pergamon Press.

Moffat, A. C. (1980), Forensic pharmacognosy – poisoning with plants, *Journal of Forensic Science Society*, **20**, 103.

Rechcigl, M. (Ed.) (1983) *Handbook of Naturally Occurring Food Toxicants*, Boca Raton: CRC Press.

Russell, F. E. and Dart, R. C. (1991) Toxic effects of animal toxins, in *Cassarett and Doull's Toxicology*, Amdur, M. O., Doull, J. and Klaassen, C. (Eds), 4th edition, New York: Pergamon Press.

Twigg, L. E. and King, D. R. (1991) The impact of fluoracetate-bearing vegetation on native Australian fauna: a review, *Oikos*, **61**, 412–430.

Wedin, G. P. (1993) Poisons of animal origin, in *General and Applied Toxicology*, Ballantyne, B., Marrs, T. and Turner, P. (Eds), Basingstoke, UK: Macmillan.

Chapter 10

Household Products

Introduction

This group of potential poisons comprises many substances, some of which fit into one or more of the other categories already discussed. For example, the herbicide paraquat (see Chapter 7) is widely used by domestic gardeners as well as by horticulturalists, and consequently it is often found in the home. Drugs too are often found around the household, however, these have been discussed already and will not be further mentioned.

Household products feature in poisoning cases usually after accidental ingestion by children and occasionally in suicide cases. The majority of enquiries relating to childhood poisoning, especially in children under 5-years-old, are in connection with non-medicinal, mainly household products or toxic substances to which people may be exposed in the home. However, the number of deaths due to substances used in the home is small, six in the UK in 1978 and 21 in the USA in 1976. The majority of deaths in children under 10-years of age are due to carbon monoxide and consequently this will be discussed in detail.

Some of the potentially toxic substances found in the home are corrosive and some are generally only ingested intentionally. Bleach is perhaps the substance most commonly involved in poisoning cases. Other substances include strong detergents such as dishwasher powder, drain cleaners which are generally caustic (i.e. corrosive), and kettle descalers which are corrosive (Figure 10.1). When bleach is ingested orally it causes burning to the throat, mouth and oesophagus. The tissue damage results in oedema in the pharynx and larynx. In the stomach the presence of endogenous hydrochloric acid generates hypochlorous acid which is an irritant, and chlorine gas which may be inhaled causing toxic effects in, and damage to, the lungs. However, serious injury from ingestion of bleach rarely occurs as it requires relatively large quantities and this is usually intentional rather than accidental.

Hydrocarbon solvents such as turpentine substitute and white spirit are often used for cleaning paint brushes. They may be dangerous by aspiration which can lead to a chemical pneumonitis. Having a low viscosity and being volatile, the solvent spreads through the lungs easily and therefore can affect a large area.

AYLESBURY PLUS, WEDNESDAY, SEPTEMBER 16 1987

Agonising death of haunted woman

A HAUNTED Wendover woman died an agonising death after drinking kettle descaler.

In the last year Mrs Heidi Mason, 44, of Orchard Close, Wendover, had tried to kill herself with pill overdoses, a razor blade and a plastic bag after becoming a victim of serious depression.

She was found, bleeding from the mouth, half-conscious but dying, in the grounds of St John's psychiatric hospital, Stone, where she was a voluntary patient, on June 4.

Her stomach was almost entirely eaten away by the acid and her mouth and throat badly blistered.

But despite her history of suicide attempts, Bucks coroner Rodney Corner refused to record a verdict of suicide at Mrs Mason's inquest in Aylesbury on Friday.

He recorded an open verdict, saying he could not be certain she had intended to kill herself this time.

Dr Julian Candy, psychologist at St John's, told the inquest that Mrs Mason believed that people around her knew certain things about her past.

'Mrs Mason suffered from self-blame, guilt and depression, and discussed suicide with me on several occasions,' said Dr Candy.

'She had an intense feeling of hopelessness. A number of deaths in the family including her mother's and stepfather's caused her great distress.'

Pathologist Dr Andrew Tudway said that Mrs Mason's stomach was almost entirely corroded and her mouth and throat ulcerated by the formic acid in the kettle descaler.

Figure 10.1. A headline reminds us of the potential toxicity of household substances. In this case, kettle descaler containing corrosive formic acid was taken intentionally.
Taken from the newspaper, *Aylesbury Plus*, 16 September 1987, with permission.

Carbon Monoxide

This highly toxic gas is still a major cause of poisoning deaths in the UK despite the fact that a major source, coal gas, has been replaced by natural gas. Several hundred deaths occur annually and carbon monoxide poisoning is still the major cause of death from poisoning in children. The gas is found in car exhausts and results from the inefficient burning of hydrocarbon fuels in engines as well as in stoves and boilers especially where there is poor ventilation. There have, in fact, been a number of poisonings recently, some with fatal outcomes which have been highlighted in the press and on television in the UK. In one recent case, a birds nest had blocked the chimney of a holiday cottage and so when the fire was lit, the lack of ventilation caused the fire to produce carbon monoxide. All the members of the family subsequently died in the house from carbon monoxide poisoning (see Emsley, Bibliography).

Carbon monoxide is a very simple poison and its mode of action has been understood for many years. Poisoning with it is also relatively simple to treat. In 1895 Haldane conducted experiments with carbon monoxide using himself as a subject. He carefully documented the effects as the concentration of carbon monoxide in his blood stream rose towards lethal levels. Through his studies and the earlier work of Claude Bernard in 1865 we now know much about the mechanism of action of carbon monoxide as a poison.

Carbon monoxide reacts with the haemoglobin in red blood cells. It does this by binding to the iron atom of the haem molecule in the same way as oxygen (Figure 10.2). Carbon monoxide binds more avidly than oxygen, however, and the resulting haemoglobin cannot carry out its normal function of transporting oxygen. Therefore, there is competition for binding to haemoglobin between oxygen and carbon monoxide and the concentration of the latter is a crucial factor. As carbon monoxide binds much more avidly to the

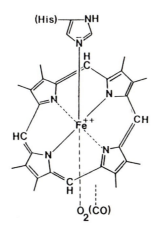

Figure 10.2. The haem moiety of the haemoglobin molecule showing the binding of the oxygen molecule to the iron atom. As shown in the diagram, carbon monoxide (CO) binds at the same site as the oxygen molecule, but it is bound much more tightly. (His is the side chain of the amino acid Histidine.)

iron atom the concentration of the toxic gas necessary to saturate the haemoglobin is much less than that of oxygen in air. This was determined by Haldane and is shown by his equation:

$$\frac{[COHb]}{[HbO_2]} = \frac{M[P_{CO}]}{[P_{O2}]}$$

where M is 220, at pH 7.4 in man. [COHb] and [HbO$_2$] are the concentration of carboxyhaemoglobin and haemoglobin respectively. [P$_{CO}$] and [P$_{O2}$] are the partial pressures of carbon monoxide and oxygen respectively.

Consequently, for 50 per cent saturation of haemoglobin with carbon monoxide, where 50 per cent of the haemoglobin in the blood is carboxy-haemoglobin, the concentration of carbon monoxide need only be 1/220 of that of oxygen in the air or about 0.1 per cent. A level of 50 per cent carboxy-haemoglobin would certainly be lethal for a human after a relatively short time. As carbon monoxide is also odourless and tasteless, it is an extremely dangerous poison. The result of carbon monoxide poisoning is that the tissues are starved of oxygen and suffer ischaemic damage. Energy production is reduced, only anaerobic respiration being possible and, hence, there is an accumulation of lactic acid causing acidosis.

The symptoms of carbon monoxide poisoning depend on the concentration to which the victim is exposed. There is often headache, mental confusion, agitation, nausea and vomiting. The skin becomes characteristically pink due to the carboxyhaemoglobin in the blood. The victim hyperventilates and will eventually lose consciousness and suffer respiratory failure. There may be brain and cardiac damage resulting from the hypoxia, and also cardiac arrythmias and other malfunctions of the heart can occur.

Treatment is relatively simple, especially for mild cases and involves removing the victim from the source of carbon monoxide, or causing fresh uncontaminated air to be introduced into the immediate environment. As the

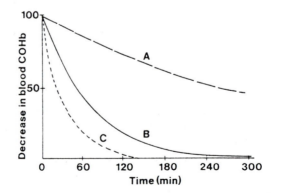

Figure 10.3. The dissociation of carboxyhaemoglobin in the bloodstream of a patient poisoned with carbon monoxide. The graphs show the effects of breathing air (A), oxygen (B) or oxygen at increased pressure (2.5 atmospheres) (C) on the rate of dissociation.
Data from Meredith, T. J. and Vale, J. A. (1981), Antidotes, pp. 33–45, Figure 5.9, in *Poisoning-Diagnosis and Treatment*, J. A. Vale and T. J. Meredith (Eds), London: Update Books.

concentration of carbon monoxide in the ambient air and hence the inspired air falls, the carboxyhaemoglobin dissociates and the carbon monoxide is expired. This rate of loss of carbon monoxide from the blood (half-life around 250 minutes) can be increased by making the patient breathe oxygen rather than air (half-life reduced to 50 minutes). For severe poisoning cases the use of oxygen at elevated pressures (2.5 atmospheres) will reduce the half-life of elimination to around 22 minutes (Figure 10.3). The reductions in half-life with oxygen at elevated concentrations and pressures can be predicted from the Haldane equation.

Antifreeze: Ethylene Glycol

Antifreeze liquid contains one or sometimes two toxic compounds which may feature in poisoning, either accidental or suicidal. The major constituent of antifreeze is ethylene glycol but this may sometimes be combined with methanol.

Ethylene glycol is a dihydric alcohol and a sweet tasting liquid, which has effects on the state of mind similar to those of ethanol. It may sometimes be consumed instead of normal alcohol by alcoholics. It is very toxic, however, and fatal poisoning may occur after as little as a cupful of antifreeze.

It is not intrinsically toxic but requires metabolism. There are various intermediate metabolic products terminating in oxalic acid (Figure 2.13). The intermediate acidic metabolites cause acidosis directly and also by increasing the level of NADH which is then utilized in the production of lactic acid. As well as being acidic, oxalic acid damages the brain by crystallizing there. Calcium oxalate crystals may also form in the kidney tubules and cause damage.

The first step in the metabolism of ethylene glycol involves the enzyme alcohol dehydrogenase and this provides the key to the treatment of poisoning. The preferred substrate for this enzyme is ethanol and so when ethanol is present *in vivo* it is preferentially metabolized. The metabolism of ethylene glycol is therefore blocked. The treatment for ethylene glycol poisoning is, therefore, administration of ethanol (whisky or some similar spirit in an emergency) by mouth or pure ethanol can be infused intravenously until all of the ethylene glycol has been excreted from the body. Haemoperfusion or haemodialysis may also be used to remove ethylene glycol from the body.

The Austrian wine scandal of 1986 involved ethylene glycol being used to sweeten the wine. The amounts used however would not have been acutely toxic although the chronic toxic effects of ethylene glycol, deposition of calcium oxalate kidney stones, might have been a cause for concern. The fact that wine also contains ethanol raises the interesting possibility that the toxicity would be reduced by the continued presence of the antidote!

Methanol, which may sometimes be present in antifreeze, is also found in methylated spirits (industrial spirit). It is also very toxic due to its metabolism to formaldehyde and formic acid:

$$CH_3OH \rightarrow HCHO \rightarrow HCOOH$$

The former may cause blindness if the dose of methanol is not rapidly fatal. Again, as methanol is metabolized by alcohol dehydrogenase, treatment of poisoning involves administration of ethanol and correction of metabolic acidosis, in the same way as for ethylene glycol poisoning. It may be that the presence of large amounts of ethanol in methylated spirits confers some protection on those unfortunates who drink it either accidentally or intentionally as a substitute for alcoholic drinks.

Alcohol

Ethanol is perhaps our most ubiquitous drug and features in far more cases of poisoning or adverse effects than more notorious drugs such as heroin or cocaine. Many members of the general public probably do not consider alcohol to be a drug but it has both pharmacological and toxic effects. The effects of ethanol vary with the dose and there is some evidence that it may even have beneficial effects at low doses (see Saul, Bibliography). Ethanol is rapidly absorbed from the gut and distributes into body water. About 90 per cent is metabolized to acetaldehyde, acetic acid and then carbon dioxide and water at a rate of $10-20$ ml hr^{-1}. After acute doses the major effect of ethanol is depression of the central nervous system. The pharmacological effects may be desirable if the dose is low but after higher doses the effects become exaggerated, progressing through increasing visual impairment, muscular incoordination and slowed reaction times and after large, toxic doses unconsciousness and death. A lethal dose in an adult is between 300 and 500 ml (equivalent to about a litre of whisky) if taken in less than an hour. Large doses may cause a reversible change in the liver known as fatty liver where triglycerides accumulate in the hepatic cells. The effects of ethanol can be related to the plasma level and range from mild intoxication at levels of between 500 and 1500 mg l^{-1} to coma and death at levels of more than 5000 mg l^{-1}. At this level respiratory depression, hypotension, hypothermia and hypoglycaemia will occur. The hypoglycaemia is largely due to the inhibition of gluconeogenesis by ethanol.

After chronic exposure to ethanol the liver is the main target organ although the brain may also suffer. Cirrhosis of the liver occurs after chronic abuse of alcohol and in this toxic effect the architecture of the liver is altered by the replacement of normal tissue by collagen so that it functions less efficiently. The biochemical basis of the hepatic effects of ethanol are complex and involve alterations in the level of cofactors such as NADH and disturbances in intermediary metabolism. Thus, a shift in the redox potential with an increased NADH/NAD ratio leads to impaired mitochondrial oxidation of fatty acids such that more triglyceride is synthesized. Ethanol, however, causes various other metabolic effects which contribute to the toxicity.

Ethanol is now classified as a carcinogen from epidemiological evidence in man which associates cancer of the liver and parts of the gastrointestinal tract to its use.

Glue Sniffing and Solvent Abuse

Glue sniffing and solvent abuse became common among teenagers during the 1970s and 1980s. Many different types of solvent were used with correspondingly different effects. Toluene is a solvent commonly found in glues and mainly causes narcosis. Some of the halogenated solvents such as those used as aerosol propellants are more hazardous, as they may cause sensitization of the myocardium to catecholamines leading to ventricular arrhythmias. This effect can lead to sudden death from heart attack, especially under certain conditions such as fright, and over 120 deaths occurred in the UK in 1991. Solvents are found in many different household products including glues, paints, paint strippers, aerosols, varnishes, cleaning fluids and fire extinguishers and so the scope for abuse is enormous. The acute toxic effects of solvents are mainly narcosis or anaesthesia and the more serious sensitization of the heart. The chronic effects are in many cases unknown but may include changes in personality and general morbidity. There are, however, known cases of chronic cardiac toxicity due to trichloroethane exposure.

Questions

1. Describe the mechanism of toxicity of carbon monoxide and explain how it is treated. Why is it a potentially very dangerous compound?
2. Compare and contrast the toxicology of ethylene glycol and methanol.
3. 'Ethanol is a toxic drug widely available to the general public.' Discuss this statement.

Bibliography

Backer, R. C. (1993) Forensic toxicology: a broad overview of general principles, in *General and Applied Toxicology*, Ballantyne, B., Marrs, T. and Turner, P. (Eds), Basingstoke, UK: Macmillan.

Dreisbach, R. H. (1983), *Handbook of Poisoning: Diagnosis and Treatment*, 11th edition, Los Altos: C. A. Lange.

Ellenhorn, M. J. and Barceloux, D. G. (1988) *Medical Toxicology. Diagnosis and Treatment of Human Poisoning*, New York: Elsevier.

Emsley, J. Silent killer in the air we breathe, *The Independent*, 1993.

Flanagan, R. J., Widdop, B., Ramsey, J. D. and Loveland, M. (1988) Analytical toxicology, *Human Toxicology*, **7**, 489–502.

Polson, C. J., Green, M. A. and Lee, M. R. (1983) *Clinical Toxicology*, London: Pitman.

Rumack, B. H. and Lovejoy, F. H. (1991) Clinical toxicology, in *Cassarett and Doull's Toxicology*, Amdur, M. O., Doull, J. and Klaassen, C. (Eds), 4th edition, New York: Pergamon Press.

Saul, H. (1994) The debate over the limits, *New Scientists*, 1932, 12–13.

Chapter 11

Toxicity Testing and Risk Assessment

Introduction

In most industrialized countries, drugs (including veterinary medicines), food additives and contaminants, industrial chemicals, pesticides and cosmetics, to which humans and other living organisms in the environment may be exposed, have to be tested for toxicity. The regulations can vary between countries, however, and it is not within the scope of this book to discuss the regulations in any detail. More detail of the regulations may be gained from the references in the Bibliography. The purpose of Regulatory Toxicology is to ensure that the benefits of chemical substances intended for use by humans outweigh the risks from that use.

The conduct of the toxicity tests required depends partly on the type of substance and its expected use and also on the regulations of the particular country. The amount of data necessary also depends on the end use of the substance. For instance, industrial chemicals produced in small quantities may require only minimal toxicity data whereas drugs to be administered to humans require extensive toxicological testing. Pesticides may have to be tested for their effects on many different types of animal and plant in the environment and examined for their persistence.

Toxicity tests all share certain basic principles. They usually involve exposing experimental animals or plants to the test substance under controlled conditions. For existing chemicals, however, toxicological information may also be obtained from humans and animals such as those given drugs during clinical trials, individuals exposed in the work place and humans and other animals exposed in the general environment. Such epidemiological evidence can be extremely important.

Thus, the monitoring of exposure by measuring substances and their metabolites in body fluids and using biochemical indices of pathological change may be carried out in humans during potential exposure (see Detection of toxic responses, Chapter 3). An example is the monitoring of agricultural workers for exposure to organophosphorus compounds by measuring the degree of inhibition of cholinesterases in blood samples. Studying particular populations of predatory birds and measuring certain parameters, such as eggshell thickness and pesticide level, is an example of testing for toxicity in the field.

For human and veterinary medicines in the UK there is a system for reporting adverse reactions to drugs: for human medicines this is the yellow card system; for veterinary drugs adverse reactions of both the animal patient and the human user are reported. Data relating to exposure is vitally important in the eventual assessment of the whole toxicological database for a particular compound.

Pesticides and other chemical substances which can contaminate the environment will also need to be examined for their persistence in the environment and their behaviour in food chains. The stability of such compounds in particular environments is also of importance. Consequently, ecotoxicology involves more extensive residue analysis than does drug toxicology for example. The exceptions to this are veterinary medicines where the estimation of residues in animals intended for human consumption is vitally important.

Examples of pertinent questions which should be asked before any toxicity study are:

1. is it a novel compound or has it been in use for some time?;
2. is it to be released into the environment?;
3. is it to be added to human food?;
4. is it to be given as a single dose or repeatedly?;
5. at what dosage level is it to be administered?;
6. what age group will be exposed?;
7. are pregnant women or women of childbearing age likely to be exposed?.

Toxicity may be an intrinsic property of a molecule which results from interaction with a particular biological system. Consequently, a knowledge of the physico-chemical properties of that molecule may help the toxicologist to understand the toxicity or potential toxicity and to predict the likely disposition and metabolism. Indeed, we have seen several examples in this book of the importance of physico-chemical principles in toxicology. Structure-activity relationships are beginning to be used in toxicology as they are in pharmacology, especially in the field of chemical mutagenesis\carcinogenesis. This initial knowledge from preliminary studies may also influence the course of the subsequent toxicity tests especially if there are similarities with other compounds of known toxicity. Hence, the solubility, partition coefficient, melting or boiling point, vapour pressure and purity are important parameters. For example, an industrial chemical which is a very volatile liquid (i.e. with a high vapour pressure) should at least be tested for toxicity by inhalation and possibly by skin application.

As well as physico-chemical considerations there are also biological considerations and the following are the major ones:

1. the most appropriate species to study,
2. the sex of the animals used,
3. the use of inbred or outbred strains,
4. housing,
5. diet,

6. animal health,
7. metabolic similarity to man,
8. the route of administration,
9. duration of the toxicity study,
10. the numbers of animals used,
11. vehicle.

The route of administration and vehicle will depend on the expected end use or, if a drug for example, on the means of administration. The parameters to be measured may also be dependent on the particular study. For example, metabolic studies can be combined with a toxicity study and plasma levels measured as well as urinary metabolites identified and clinical chemical parameters studied. The biochemical and pathological measurements to be made will also be decided before the study is started.

Initial toxicity studies will usually be carried out to determine the approximate range of toxic dosage. For a drug this may already be known from pharmacological studies but for an industrial chemical, for instance, nothing may be known of its biological activity. Consequently, the initial range-finding studies may utilize dosage on a logarithmic scale or half-log scale. These initial studies are important if large numbers of animals are not to be wasted in later studies. The initial tests will also involve observation of the animals in order to gain insight into the possible toxic effects.

Once the approximate toxic dosage range is known then various detailed toxicity studies can be carried out. These will be followed by various other toxicity tests, usually including the following: acute, sub-acute (28- or 90-day), chronic (lifetime), mutagenicity, carcinogenicity, teratogenicity, reproductive studies and *in vitro* tests. For some compounds there may also be other types of toxicity test such as irritancy and skin sensitization studies.

There are different requirements for drugs, food additives and contaminants, industrial chemicals, cosmetics and pesticides because of the different circumstances of exposure. Chemicals which are to be used in the environment, such as pesticides and industrial chemicals which might be accidently released into the environment, will also undergo ecotoxicity tests. These will include tests with invertebrates such as *Daphnia*, earthworms, fish, phytoplankton and higher plants.

Acute Toxicity Tests

Acute toxicity tests are those designed to determine the effects which occur within a short period after dosing. These tests can determine a dose-response relationship and the LD_{50} value. The exact conduct of toxicity studies will vary depending on the compound, its eventual use and the particular regulations to be satisfied. Usually at least four dosages are used which may be in logarithmic progression especially if no range-finding studies have been done. Although the traditional LD_{50} determination is now less popular with many toxicologists it is still required by some regulatory authorities. (For more information on

Table 11.1. Investigation of acute oral toxicity and estimation of maximum non-lethal oral dosage for classification purposes.

Test dosage	Result	Action/classification
5 mg kg^{-1}	<90% survival	*Very toxic*
	>90% survival but toxicity	*Toxic*
	>90% survival no toxicity	Retest at 50 mg kg^{-1}
50 mg kg^{-1}	<90% survival	*Toxic*; test/retest at 5 mg kg^{-1}
	>90% survival but toxicity	*Harmful*
	>90% survival no toxicity	Retest at 500 mg kg^{-1}
500 mg kg^{-1}	<90% survival or toxicity	*Harmful*; test/retest at 50 mg kg^{-1}
	>90% survival no toxicity	*Unclassified*

This table has been adapted from M. J. van den Heuvel *et al.*, Human Toxicology, 6, 279, 1987.

this test see the publications in the Bibliography.) Recently an alternative to this test which attempts to find the approximate toxic dosage but uses far fewer animals has been suggested by the British Toxicology Society. In this procedure a small number of animals, such as five of each sex, are exposed to the chemical under test at a dosage level of 5 mg kg^{-1} (for example) and observed for signs of toxicity. If 90 per cent or more of the animals survive without signs of toxicity then a larger dosage, such as 50 mg kg^{-1} is employed. If again 90 per cent or more survive without signs of toxicity then the chemical is termed unclassified. Depending on the dosage required for toxicity to be evident then the chemical can be classified as shown in Table 11.1.

The information to be gained from an acute toxicity test is the nature of the dose-response relationship and observations on the toxic effects and time to death, if any of the animals die. The LD$_{50}$ value may also be determined if sufficient animals at each dosage level have been used. It is important that the dosage range used is wide enough for toxic effects to be manifested at the highest dosages used unless this would require doses that were unrealistic in relation to the expected dose or exposure. The dosage range and the method of administration will be influenced by the expected or intended route of administration and likely dosage or exposure concentration.

At the end of the toxicity test the surviving animals are killed and undergo a post-mortem with a pathological examination of tissues. Animals dying during the study should also undergo a post-mortem.

Sub-Acute Toxicity Tests

Following acute toxicity tests, sub-acute toxicity tests are usually carried out. These involve exposing the animals to the substance under test for a prolonged period, usually 28 or 90 days. The exposure is frequent and usually daily. The sub-acute tests which are also known as sub-chronic tests, provide information on the target organs affected by the compound and the major toxic effects. Toxic effects which have a slow onset can be detected and reversible and adaptive responses may become apparent during the test. Measurements of levels of the compound in blood and tissues can be made and this information correlated with any toxic effects seen. At the end of the study pathological examination is carried out and during the study clinical chemical measurements should indicate the development of any pathological lesions. The data derived from sub-acute toxicity studies also help in the design of chronic toxicity studies. Attempts are usually made in sub-acute toxicity studies to identify a no-observed effect level, taking data from other tests into consideration.

Chronic Toxicity Tests

These tests involve lifetime exposure of animals to the compound of interest. As with sub-acute toxicity tests the chronic toxicity test will terminate with a pathological examination and there may also be clinical chemical measurements made throughout at intervals. These clinical chemical measurements can indicate the development of pathological changes which can then be detected at post-mortem. Changes in other simple measurements such as body weight and food and water intake may also indicate adverse effects. Chronic toxicity studies are important for drugs administered over long periods of time, for food additives to which we may be exposed for our whole lifetimes and for environmental and industrial chemicals where we may be exposed to low levels for long periods.

For all three types of toxicity test, selection of dosages, species, strain of animal, route of exposure, parameters measured and many other considerations are vitally important. These considerations will clearly be influenced by the particular type of chemical, expected circumstances of exposure and the regulations of the countries in which the substance is to be used. For details of these toxicity tests the reader is referred to the texts given in the Bibliography.

The requirements of the New Substances Regulations in the UK serve to illustrate the range of physico-chemical, toxicological and ecotoxicological studies that may be required. Under these regulations the amount of testing required depends upon the amount of the substance produced but the minimum requirements are shown in Table 11.2. In addition, teratology, fertility, further subchronic, carcinogenicity and chronic toxicity studies may be required depending on the amount of the compound produced and the results of other tests. It may also be necessary to repeat some of the studies already carried out but using alternative routes of administration or a different species of animal for instance. Similarly ecotoxicology studies may also need to be increased to include prolonged toxicity studies in *Daphnia* and fish, effects on higher plants and determination of bioaccumulation in fish and possibly other species. The tests described are the basic ones required and serve to illustrate the principles involved. However, other tests will also be required such as teratogenicity and other reproductive studies, carcinogenicity, mutagenicity, irritancy and skin sensitization.

Table 11.2. Summary of major information required for a new chemical substance[*].

Identity	**Toxicology studies**
name/trade name	acute toxicity (oral/inhalation/cutaneous)
formulae (empirical/structural)	skin and eye irritancy
composition	skin sensitization
methods of detection/determination	subacute toxicity (28 days)
	mutagenicity (bacterial and non-bacterial)
Uses and Precautions	**Ecotoxicological studies**
proposed uses	toxicity to fish
estimated production/importation	toxicity to *Daphnia*
handling/storage/transport methods and	degradation data (BOD, BOD/COD)
precautions	
emergency measures	
Physico-chemical properties	**Possibility of rendering substances harmless**
melting point	for industry
boiling point	for public
relative density	declaration concerning the possibility of
	unfavourable effects
vapour pressure	proposed classification and labelling
surface tension	proposals for any recommended precautions
	for safe use
water solubility	
fat solubility	
partition coefficient (octanol/water)	
flash point	
flammability	
explosive properties	
auto-flammability	
oxidizing properties	

[*] This represents the minimal information required for a new substance under the UK and EC regulations. Taken from *Medical Information* (1985) **10**, 123–127, Woodward and Tomlinson.

Reproductive studies determine the effect of the compound on the reproductive process. Thus, teratogenicity tests examine the effect of the compound on the development of the embryo and foetus. These may be detected as gross anatomical abnormalities in the new born animal or may be more subtle effects such as changes in behaviour. The effect of the compound on the fertility of both male and female animals may also be determined in reproductive toxicity tests. Data from other tests may also be relevant, such as pathological evidence of testicular damage which might additionally be detected as a decrease in male fertility.

Mutagenicity tests determine whether the compound has potential to cause genetic damage and so induce a mutation in germ cells and somatic cells. Such tests indicate whether a compound may have the potential to induce cancers. Mutagenicity tests are carried out in bacteria and cultured mammalian cells *in vitro*. *In vivo* assays include the micronucleus test and the dominant lethal assay (see Bibliography for details).

Carcinogenicity tests may also be required, especially if the mutagenicity tests are positive. The compound is given for the life time of the animal, administered either in the drinking water or diet. The appearance of tumours at post-mortem or perhaps before the animal dies are detected from histopathological studies of sections of tissues from the major organs.

Irritancy and skin sensitization tests may also be required, especially for industrial chemicals and pesticides. Irritancy tests are usually carried out on rabbit skin or eyes. The skin sensitization test is normally carried out in the guinea pig and a positive result indicates that the compound has the potential to cause contact dermatitis in humans. Some compounds may also cause pulmonary sensitization but there is no reliable animal model for this effect. Consideration of the toxicity data may suggest that further studies be carried out, such as an investigation to show that an effect is peculiar to a particular species and therefore not relevant to man.

Toxicity tests are normally either carried out by the company producing the compound or a contract research laboratory or a combination of both. The conduct of the toxicity and ecotoxicity studies should conform to certain guidelines, such as those issued by the Organisation for Economic Cooperation and Development (OECD). These guidelines are often enshrined in national regulatory requirements such as those in the UK and USA. Toxicity tests also now must be carried out in compliance with a system known as Good Laboratory Practice (GLP), which governs every aspect of the conduct of studies including the reporting of results. This system was introduced to ensure that toxicity tests are competently carried out and that data is not fabricated, following a notorious situation which arose in the USA.

As well as the requirements of regulatory agencies toxicity data may also have other uses. Indeed, the data may be life saving in cases of human and animal poisoning. For example, animal studies on cyanide toxicity provided data which was useful in the treatment of poisoning with cyanide. The absence of any toxicity data on methylisocyanate probably hampered the efforts of rescue workers and clinicians at Bhopal in India after the massive disaster where methylisocyanate leaked from a chemical plant there. Basic studies on paracetamol toxicity led directly to the use of an antidote which has proved extremely successful and life saving. Attempts to understand the mechanisms underlying the toxicity of compounds will allow better prediction of toxicity and also better design of tests to discover toxic potential.

Risk Assessment and Interpretation of Toxicological Data

At least 65 000 chemicals are currently produced in the USA with 500–1000 new chemicals added each year. In the past, perhaps chemicals were too readily produced and used without due care and attention. Rachel Carson in her book, *Silent Spring* showed the risks of such actions. The general public is now very suspicious of all chemicals and there is perhaps an exaggerated fear of poisoning from chemicals in the environment and a belief that all chemicals are hazardous. Regulation has been introduced in many countries in response to this public fear and pressure. Clearly regulation is necessary, but where possible guidelines should be issued rather than strict rules for the assessment of every case in the same way. A major problem with toxicological data is the assessment of hazards and the subsequent calculation of risks and estimation of risk versus benefit.

'Risk is a measure of the probability that an adverse effect will occur.' This may be absolute risk which is the excess risk due to exposure, or relative risk which is the ratio of risk in the exposed to the unexposed population. For a chemical being considered as a toxic hazard, risk is the expected frequency of undesirable effects arising from exposure to that chemical and is a function of the intrinsic toxicity and the dose or exposure level. The exposure level is determined by the duration, frequency and intensity of exposure, which will in turn depend on the circumstances of exposure in a particular environment. For example, in a factory manufacturing a particular chemical the production workers may suffer continuous moderate exposure whereas maintenance workers may be subject to much higher concentrations periodically during work on a reaction vessel. Workers in other parts of the factory and office workers on the site may have only negligible exposure and perhaps be only at risk from an accidental leak. Depending on the disposition and toxicity of the particular compound, the risk to the production worker with a greater total exposure may be less than that to the maintenance worker exposed to very high concentrations. Alternatively, if the compound causes allergic reactions then continuous exposure will be more important and the production worker may be more at risk. Therefore, risk assessment involves first an identification of the hazard, followed by an estimation of the exposure level and frequency, and then a knowledge of the *in vivo* disposition, toxicity and dose response relationship.

The assessment of exposure and dose is critical in risk assessment but can be very difficult to estimate in a human population as exposure may be affected by many factors. For instance, lifestyle varies among humans, the exposure may vary in frequency and it may be periodic. Such factors are difficult to simulate. In manufacturing plants the workers may be monitored for exposure to a substance by measuring its concentration in their blood or urine. Alternatively their exposure may be monitored by the use of personal or environmental metering systems.

In the general population, however, this is much more difficult. So although currently available analytical methods are often able to very accurately determine minute levels of toxic compounds in the environment, determination of the exposure of humans to those compounds is much more difficult and much less precise.

The accuracy of measurement has increased over the years and so has our ability to detect ever smaller amounts but this may lead to paranoia over insignificant levels of substances.

The science of toxicology involves observing the qualitative and quantitative effects of compounds in biological systems *in vivo* and *in vitro*. The art of toxicology is the use of this data or a limited database to predict the likelihood or probability of occurrence of a toxic effect. This requires extrapolation between species and between doses or levels of exposure.

Acute toxic effects are usually easier to deal with than chronic toxic effects as it is generally accepted that there will be a 'no observed adverse effect level' or NOAEL. This can be derived from the dose-response relationship. So it is possible to derive an acceptable daily intake value or ADI for a food additive, for example, a therapeutic index in the case of a drug or a TLV (MEL) for an industrial chemical (see Chapter 2 or Glossary for a definition of these terms). Chronic toxicity and especially carcinogenicity and teratogenicity are more difficult to deal with. Theoretically, a single 'hit' or reaction of a compound or its metabolite on the crucial part of one DNA molecule might be sufficient to initiate a cancerous change. However, the chances of one molecule reaching this target site are probably small for most compounds. This will be determined by the potency, absorption, distribution and metabolism of the compound and these will affect its ability to reach and damage DNA. The capacity of the particular cell to repair such damage will also be crucial. Effectively, therefore, there may be a threshold dose for a carcinogen but it is difficult to determine in mammals *in vivo* because the crucial biochemical changes at the cellular level are currently difficult if not impossible to detect. Consequently, bacterial assays such as the Ames test are used which detect such mutagenic changes. The results from animal carcinogenicity testing studies are particularly hard to assess as it is necessary but difficult to show an increased frequency of tumours in a small population such as those used in animal cancer studies, in which there may already be a significant incidence of some types of tumours. There is a practical, statistical limit which determines the incidence or frequency of occurrence of a cancer which can be detected. For example, using 1000 animals it is necessary for more than five animals to be affected by cancer for the effect to be detected at the 99 per cent confidence level; but an incidence of five cases in 1000 test animals if extrapolated to man would translate into over 1 million cases of cancer in a population the size of that of the US. To use even larger numbers of animals would be impractical, extremely expensive, and challenged on ethical (animal rights) grounds. So assessing cancer risk from carcinogenicity studies is very difficult and those conducting and assessing the tests tend to err on the side of caution. One way around the dilemma of low incidence is to increase the doses used in the animal tests on the assumption that the dose-response is linear and so extrapolation backwards is possible. This has given rise to various models but estimates from these models vary; the precision of the mathematical model is largely irrelevant if the quality of the original toxicological data is poor. There may be large margins of error and uncertainty. Unfortunately the public may take the exposure limits and similar data issued at face value or alternately disbelieve them completely. Consequently, doses close to the Maximum Tolerated Dose (MTD) are used in carcinogenicity testing despite the problems of dose-dependent metabolism, dose-dependent kinetics, and the possibility of other pathological effects influencing the carcinogenicity. This approach is contentious, however, as carcinogens may show dose dependent metabolism and with weak or equivocal carcinogens such as saccharin (see Chapter 6) and especially non-genotoxic carcinogens this may be crucial to the interpretation of the carcinogenicity data. That is, large doses of a compound may be metabolized in a quantitatively or qualitatively different manner to that of the expected dose or exposure level. Consequently, a compound may only be carcinogenic under those extreme dosing conditions. For example, the industrial chemical hydrazine is a weak carcinogen after high exposure or dose levels. It also causes DNA methylation, a possibly mutagenic event which might lead to cancer but this methylation only occurs after large, hepatotoxic doses. The implications of this are that the acute toxic effect is in some way involved in the DNA methylation and that also the acute effect is necessary for the development of the cancer.

Extrapolation between species is also a problem in risk assessment and the interpretation of toxicological data. For example, one question that arises is 'which species is the extrapolation to be made from, the most sensitive or the one which in terms of response or disposition of the compound is the most similar to man?' The species or strain used in a particular carcinogenicity study may have a high natural incidence of a specific type or types of tumour. The assessment of the significance of an increase in the incidence of this tumour and its relevance to man can pose particular problems. Therefore, risk assessment from carcinogenicity is fraught with difficulties, possibly more than any other type of toxic effect.

For acute toxic effects the dose response is often clear cut and allows a NOAEL to be estimated. However, the biology of the toxicity study must always be taken into account and a too exaggerated reliance on statistics must be avoided. Because of the problems of interspecies extrapolation and interpretation of low incidences of tumours, risk assessment may give rise to widely disparate quantitative values. For example, for saccharin the expected number of bladder cancer cases in the USA over a 70-year period due to daily exposure to 120 mg was estimated as between 0.22 and 1.144×10^6! Therefore, in the risk assessment of a particular compound other factors become important such as the likely and reasonable human exposure but in the USA the strict rules of the Delaney clause make this difficult (see Glossary for definition of Delaney Clause).

The incidence of a toxic effect may be measured under precise laboratory conditions but extrapolation to a real life situation to give an estimate of risk involves many assumptions and gives rise to uncertainties. The risk assessor has to decide which are plausible answers to questions when in reality there are either no scientific answers or these answers are obscure. Risk assessment involves questions such as which model of the dose-response curve to use for extrapolation. Pharmacokinetic, mechanistic and metabolic data will all affect this.

How should the real human exposure be estimated from limited data? The problems of doing this tend to lead to the worst case estimate and so estimates of risk will tend to exaggerate the risk to human health.

For a new chemical substance human data is not available and toxic effects in man cannot be verified by direct experiment and so extrapolation from the results of animal studies is essential. Of course the objective is to have as large a margin of safety as possible. However when there is conflicting data does one use the single positive result or the 'weight' of all the data? Inflated estimates of exposure may occur. Epidemiology may be useful for compounds that have been used for some time. Indeed, many compounds have never undergone a full range of toxicity tests (an estimated 70 per cent in USA) and it would clearly be an enormous task to test all such compounds. Consequently, a reliance on epidemiology is unavoidable.

Risk assessment is followed by risk management and this includes a consideration of the benefits which inevitably involves politics and economics. Risk assessment itself may also be influenced by these factors.

Conclusions

As yet, toxicologists only partially understand the mechanisms underlying relatively few toxic effects of chemicals. Consequently the assessment of risk to man will remain difficult and uncertain. The limitations need to be borne in mind by the public, by industrialists, economists and regulatory officials, but also by toxicologists themselves.

Perhaps the public expects too much from scientists in general and toxicologists in particular. Toxicology cannot provide all of the answers the public often demands as they are beyond current science. The public may demand absolute safety but this is an impossible dream. One of the duties of the toxicologist is to make sure the limitations are understood.

Perhaps the real crux of the problem of interpretation of toxicological data in the light of increasing and widespread exposure of humans to chemicals is the assessment of risk versus benefit. Although the public may not always be aware of the fact that chemicals confer benefits on society, and that there is a greater or lesser risk attached to their use, the benefits may be hard to quantify and compare with the risk. However, just as we take a quantifiable risk when we drive a car because its use is convenient and maybe essential, then we should apply similar principles to the chemicals we use. Unfortunately the risks and benefits may not always be equally shared, with one section of society reaping financial benefits while another risks the adverse effects.

Questions

1. What factors need to be taken into account when designing safety evaluation studies?
2. Write short notes on the following:

   (a) acute toxicity tests;
   (b) sub-acute toxicity tests;
   (c) chronic toxicity tests.

3. Discuss the difficulties inherent in the interpretation of toxicological data for risk assessment.

Bibliography

Ballantyne, B., Marrs, T. and Turner, P. (Eds) (1993) Regulatory toxicology, part six, vol. 2, *General and Applied Toxicology*, Basingstoke, UK: Macmillan.
Griffin, J. P. (1985) Predictive value of animal toxicity studies, *ATLA*, **12**, 163.

Hayes, A. W. (Ed.) (1989) *Principles and Methods of Toxicology*, 2nd edition, New York: Raven Press.

Heuvel, M. J. Van Den, Dayan, A. D. and Shillaker, R. O. (1987) Evaluation of the BTS approach to the testing of substances and preparations for their acute toxicity, *Human Toxicology*, **6**, 279.

Homburger, F. (Ed.) (1983–) *Safety Evaluation and Regulation of Chemicals*, 3 vols, Basel: Karger.

Lu, F. C. (1991) *Basic Toxicology*, 2nd edition, Washington, DC: Hemisphere.

Merrill, R. A. (1991) Regulatory toxicology, in *Cassarett and Doull's Toxicology*, Amdur, M. O., Doull, J. and Klaassen, C. (Eds), 4th edition, New York: Pergamon Press.

NIEHS (1987), Basic research in risk assessment, *Environmental Health Perspectives*, **76** (Dec).

Roberts, C. N. (Ed.) (1989) *Risk Assessment – The Common Ground*, Eye, Suffolk: Life Science Research.

Roloff, M. V. (Ed.) (1987) *Human Risk Assessment. The Role of Animal Selection and Extrapolation*, Philadelphia: Taylor & Francis.

Scala, R. A. (1991) Risk assessment, in *Cassarett and Doull's Toxicology*, Amdur, M. O., Doull, J. and Klaassen, C. (Eds), 4th edition, New York: Pergamon Press.

Wilkinson, C. F. (1986) Risk assessment and regulatory policy, *Comments on Toxicology*, **1**, 1–21.

Zbindon, G. and Flury-Reversi, M. (1981) Significance of the LD_{50} test for the toxicological evaluation of chemical substances, *Archives of Toxicology*, **47**, 77.

Glossary

Acidosis/alkalosis The condition when the pH of the blood falls/rises outside the normal acceptable limits.

Acid rain The deposition of acids (sulphuric and nitric) in rain and also the dry deposition of sulphur dioxide and nitrogen oxides.

Acute Short term exposure or response.

Additive When the toxic effect of a mixture is equal to the sum of the toxicities of the components.

ADI The Acceptable Daily Intake. 'The daily intake of a chemical which during an entire lifetime appears to be without appreciable risk on the basis of all the known facts at the time.'

Aerobic/anaerobic A process carried out in the presence/absence of air.

Aerosol A colloidal system with a gas as the dispersion medium (such as a fog or mist of droplets or particles).

Allergic reaction A reaction to a foreign agent giving rise to a hypersensitive state, mediated via an immunological mechanism and resulting in a particular series of responses.

Anaphylactic reaction A type I immunological response.

Anoxia Absence of oxygen in the tissues.

Antagonism When the toxic effect of a mixture is less than the sum of the toxicities of the components.

Antibody A protein produced by lymphoid tissue in response to, and specific for, a foreign substance or antigen.

Anticoagulant A substance which inhibits the normal process of blood clotting.

Antidote A substance which specifically blocks or reduces the action of a poison.

Antigen A protein or other macromolecule which is recognized as foreign by the immune system in an animal.

Antiport Membrane carrier system in which two substances are transported in opposite directions.

Asbestosis Damage to the lungs caused specifically by exposure to, and inhalation of, asbestos fibres.

Ataxia Failure of muscular coordination.

AUC Area under the curve when the plasma (blood) concentration of a substance is plotted against time.

β-adrenoceptors An autonomic receptor of which there are two types, β_1 and β_2.

Bioaccumulation The accumulation of a substance in a biological organism, usually due to its lipophilicity (q.v.).

Biomagnification The process whereby the concentration of a pollutant in organisms in a food chain increases towards the top of that chain. Thus the predator at the top of the food chain will have the highest concentration of pollutant.

Biomarker Indicator of exposure to or biological effect of a chemical substance in a living system.

Blood-brain barrier A description of the inability of many substances to pass from the blood to the tissues of the brain.

BOD Biochemical Oxygen Demand. This measurement indicates the ability of micro-organisms to metabolize an organic substance in the presence of oxygen and therefore the potential for depletion of oxygen by the substance.

Bronchocarcinoma Cancer of the lung.

Bronchoconstriction Constriction of the airways in the lungs due to exposure to irritant chemicals or to an immunological reaction involving release of inflammatory mediators.

Carcinogen/carcinogenic A substance/property of a substance which causes cancer when administered to an organism.

Cardiac arrythmias Abnormal beating rhythms in the heart.

Cardiac output The volume of blood pumped by the heart in one cycle.

Cerebral palsy A motor disorder due to damage to the brain.

Cholinergic stimulation Stimulation of the nerve fibres utilizing acetylcholine as a neurotransmitter.

Chronic (lifetime) Long-term exposure or response.

Cirrhosis Liver disease characterized by loss of the normal microscopic lobular structure with fibrosis and nodular regeneration. Usually the result of chronic injury to tissue.

Clearance The volume of plasma cleared of a substance in unit time.

Clinical trials The initial studies carried out with a drug in human subjects.

COD Chemical Oxygen Demand. The amount of oxygen required to oxidize the substance chemically.

COD/BOD The ratio of COD to BOD gives an indication of the biodegradability of the substance.

Collagen A fibrous protein.

Complement A series of proteins found in extracellular fluids and involved in certain immunological reactions.

Cyanosis The pathological condition where there is an excessive concentration of reduced haemoglobin in the blood.

Cytochrome a₃ A haem-containing enzyme which is part of the cytochrome c oxidase complex, the terminal cytochrome in the mitochondrial electron transport chain.

Cytological examination Examination of cells or examination for the presence of cells in urine.

Cytosol The internal part of the cell excluding the organelles.

Delaney Amendment Amendment to the Food, Drug and Cosmetic Act of the Food and Drug Administration of the United States. The amendment states that food additives which cause cancer in humans or animals at any level shall not be considered safe and are, therefore, prohibited.

Dermatitis Inflammation of the skin.

Detritivore food chain An animal which uses decaying organic matter as a food source, after the initial breakdown of the material by decomposers such as bacteria and fungi is known as a 'detritivore.' The type of food chain which relies on decaying organic matter for its primary energy source is known as a 'detritivore food chain.'

Dinoflagellates Single-celled marine algae possessing two flagella.

Disulphide bridge A sulphur-sulphur bond (S-S) such as occurs commonly in proteins.

Dominant lethal assay A test designed to detect the effects of substances on the germ cells of male animals which are exposed and then mated with untreated females. The number of dead implantations or preimplantation losses in the pregnant females are then determined. The effects are usually due to chromosome damage.

ED$_{50}$ The dose which is pharmacologically effective for 50 per cent of the population exposed to the substance *or* a 50 per cent response in a biological system which is exposed to the substance.

Electrophilic A chemical description of a substance which seeks out a group or molecular position which has a preponderance of electrons and so is negatively charged.

Encephalopathy A degenerative disease of the brain.

Endogenous Part of the internal environment of a living organism.

Enterohepatic recirculation The cycling of a substance from the blood into the liver, then into the bile and gastrointestinal tract. This is followed by re-uptake into the bloodstream from the gastrointestinal tract possibly after chemical or enzymatic breakdown.

Epidemiology The study of diseases in populations.

Epigenetic When used as a description of a carcinogen or of mechanisms of carcinogenesis this means that interaction with genetic material, such as to yield a mutation, is not involved.

ER Endoplasmic reticulum. This may be divided into rough ER with attendant ribosomes involved with protein synthesis and smooth ER where cytochrome P-450 and many other drug metabolizing enzymes are located.

Eutrophication Increased nutrient concentration in water resulting in the overgrowth of plants such as algae giving rise to a depletion of oxygen. This is followed by death and decay of all the aerobic organisms in the aqueous environment with the subsequent growth of anaerobic bacteria leading to the accumulation of toxins.

Exanthema An eruptive disease or fever.

Fatty acid An organic acid with a long aliphatic chain which may be saturated or unsaturated.

Fibrosis The formation of fibrous tissue which may be a response of tissue to injury resulting in increased amounts of collagen fibres.

Ficks Law At constant temperature the rate of diffusion of a substance across a cell membrane is proportional to the concentration gradient and the surface area.

First order process The rate of the process is proportional to the concentration of the substance.

First-pass metabolism Metabolism of a drug or other chemical during the absorption process. Typically occurs in the liver or gastrointestinal tract after oral dosing.

Food chain An imaginary chain of organisms existing in the environment in which each link of the chain feeds upon the one below and is eaten by the one above. At the bottom of the food chain are plants and bacteria, at the top are carnivores.

Free radical An atom or molecule which has an unpaired electron. They may be uncharged or charged depending on the numbers of electrons. Free radicals are usually chemically very reactive.

Genotoxic Toxic to the genetic material of an organism.

Glomerulus A functional unit of the vertebrate kidney consisting of a small bunch of capillaries projecting into a capsule (Bowmans capsule) which serves to collect the filtrate from the blood of those capillaries and direct it into the kidney tubule.

Glutathione (GSH) The tripeptide glutamyl-cysteinyl-glycine. Found in most tissue, especially the liver. Plays a major role in detoxication and cellular protection.

Glycoprotein A protein containing a carbohydrate moiety.

Good Laboratory Practice (GLP) A system of protocols (standard operating procedures) recommended to be followed so as to avoid the production of unreliable and erroneous data. Accurate record keeping and careful forethought in the design of the study are important aspects of GLP.

GSH/GSSG Reduced/oxidized glutathione.

Haemodialysis The process by which a foreign substance is removed from the blood of a poisoned patient by allowing it to diffuse across a semi-permeable membrane while the blood is pumped through a special machine.

Haemoglobinuria The presence of haemoglobin in the urine.

Haemolytic anaemia The pathological condition where red blood cells undergo uncontrolled destruction.

Haemoperfusion The process by which a foreign substance is removed from the blood of a poisoned patient by allowing it to be absorbed by activated charcoal or a resin while the blood is pumped through a special machine.

Haemorrhage The escape of blood from blood vessels.

Haemorrhagic necrosis Necrosis accompanied by bleeding.

Half-life The time taken for the concentration of a compound in a body fluid to decrease by half.

Hapten A molecule which becomes attached to a protein or other macromolecule and so renders it antigenic.

Henderson-Hasselbach equation $pH = pKa + \log A^-/HA$.

Histamine A mediator of inflammatory reactions in the body which may be part of an allergic reaction.

HLA type Histocompatability antigens on the surface of nucleated cells.

Hydrophobic/hydrophilic A substance which repels/attracts water.

Hyperkinesis Hyperactivity.

Hypoglycaemia The physiological state where there is a low blood glucose concentration.

Hypoxia The physiological state where there is a low oxygen concentration in the tissues.

Idiosyncratic In toxicology this is an adverse reaction to a chemical which occurs in a single or small number of individuals as a result of an abnormality in that individual.

Immune complex A complex of antibody(ies) and antigen(s) which may lead to pathological consequences such as inflammation or blockage of a vessel.

Initiation The first stage in the multi-stage process of carcinogenesis in which there is thought to be a chemical reaction between the carcinogen and DNA.

Interferon A macromolecule produced by the body in response to a stimulus such as an infection.

Intraperitoneal/i.p. A route of administration of a compound to an animal by direct injection into the peritoneal cavity.

Irritation/irritancy Direct injury to tissue such as the skin.

Ischaemia The condition where there is a reduced or blocked blood flow to a tissue which will lead to ischaemic tissue damage.

Isozyme/isoenzyme One of several forms of an enzyme where the different forms usually catalyze similar but distinct reactions.

Keratin A tough, fibrous protein found in the skin.

Killer lymphocyte A particular type of white blood cell involved in Type IV immunological reactions.

LD$_{50}$ The lethal dose of a compound for 50 per cent of the population of organisms exposed.

Lipid peroxidation Oxidative breakdown of lipids usually involving a free radical mechanism or active oxygen species and giving rise to reactive products which may be responsible for cellular damage.

Lipid solubility see lipophilicity.

Lipophilicity A term used to describe the ability of a substance to dissolve in, or associate with, fat and therefore living tissue. This usually applies to compounds which are non-ionized or non-polar or have a non-polar portion. Therefore high lipid solubility usually implies low water solubility.

Local toxicity Toxicity which affects only the site of application or exposure.

Macromolecule A very large molecule having a polymeric structure such as a protein or nucleic acid.

Macrophage Large phagocytic cells which are components of the reticulo-endothelial system.

Maximally Tolerated Dose (MTD) The dose of a substance which causes no more than a 10 per cent weight decrease and does not cause death or any clinical signs of toxicity which would shorten the life span of an animal exposed for 90 days.

MEL Maximum Exposure Level; maximum level of occupational exposure of workers to a chemical; term used in UK.

Mesothelioma A rare form of cancer mainly affecting the pleura and caused exclusively by exposure to certain forms of asbestos.

Methaemoglobin/methaemoglobinaemia Oxidized haemoglobin/the syndrome in which a significant amount of the haemoglobin in the blood is oxidized.

Microflora/microfauna The bacteria and other organisms inhabiting the gastrointestinal tract.

Micronucleus test A test for mutagenicity (q.v.) using red blood cell stem cells from mice. The mice are exposed to the chemical and after a suitable time period the bone marrow examined for an increase in the number of micronuclei. These are chromosome fragments resulting from spindle or centromere dysfunction.

Microsomes/microsomal The subcellular fraction containing the fragments of the smooth endoplasmic reticulum (ER) after ultracentrifugation of a homogenate of the cell.

Mitochondria The intracellular organelle in which respiration and other important metabolic reactions take place.

Monooxygenase Enzyme system (such as cytochrome P_{450}) involved in the oxidation of compounds.

Mutagen/mutagenic A substance/ a property of a substance which causes some type of mutation in the genetic material of an organism exposed to it.

Myocardium The middle and thickest layer of cardiac muscle in the heart wall.

NADH The coenzyme reduced nicotinamide adenine dinucleotide.

NADPH The coenzyme reduced nicotinamide adenine dinucleotide phosphate.

Narcosis Unconsciousness induced by exposure to a solvent or volatile liquid.

Necrosis The process of cell death within a living organism and the end result of irreversible changes following cellular injury.

Nephritis Inflammation of the kidney.

Nephron The functional unit of the kidney which produces urine. It consists of a long tubule divided into sections in which reabsorption into the bloodstream of certain solutes filtered by the glomerulus from the blood takes place.

NOAEL No Observed Adverse Effect Level. The dose or exposure level at which no adverse effect is detected in the organism.

Occlusion Constriction or blockage as of a blood vessel.

Organelle A subcellular structure such as the mitochondrion or nucleus of a cell.

Osteomalacia Softening of the bones due to impaired mineralization.

Paresthesias Abnormal sensations such as tingling.

Peripheral neuropathy Damage to nerves of the peripheral, rather than central, nervous system.

Peroxidases Enzymes which catalyze oxidation utilizing hydrogen peroxide. Found in many tissues including certain types of white blood cells (neutrophils).

Persistence When applied to a chemical substance meaning its ability to remain unchanged in the environment.

Pesticide An agent used to exterminate pests of various types. Includes insecticides, herbicides and fungicides.

Phago/pinocytosis The uptake of a solid substance (phago) or solution (pino) into a cell by invagination of the cell membrane eventually forming a vesicle inside the cell.

Pharmacodynamic Relating to the effects of drugs on living systems.

Phase 1 The term applied to the first stage of drug metabolism, commonly involving either oxidation, reduction or hydrolysis of the molecule.

Phase 2 The term applied to the second stage of drug metabolism usually involving conjugation of a functional group with a moiety available endogenously and conferring water solubility on the molecule.

Phase 3 Further metabolism of a metabolic product of a phase 2 reaction such as a glutathione conjugate.

Phenotype The expression of the genotype or genetic make-up of an organism.

Phocomelia The syndrome of having foreshortened arms and legs due to an adverse effect on the embryo such as caused by thalidomide.

Phospholipid A lipid in which one of the hydroxyl groups of glycerol or sphingosine is esterified with a phosphorylated alcohol.

pH Partition Theory This states that a foreign compound in the non-ionized state will pass across a cell membrane by passive diffusion down a concentration gradient.

Plasma Blood from which the cells have been removed by centrifugation but distinct from serum in which the blood is first allowed to clot.

Pneumonitis Inflammation of the lungs.

Polar A term used to describe a molecule which is charged or has a tendency to become polarized.

Polychlorinated biphenyls A group of compounds used industrially in which a biphenyl nucleus is substituted with various numbers of chlorine atoms.

Polypeptide A chain of amino acids joined by peptide bonds.

Portal The term applied to the venous circulation draining the tissues of the gastrointestinal tract into the liver.

Potentiation When the toxic effect of a compound is increased by a non-toxic compound.

ppb Parts per billion.

ppm Parts per million. A measure of concentration of a substance in which the units of the substance are one millionth of the units of the solvent, eg μg per g.

Prescribed disease An industrial disease which is recognized as such for the purposes of compensation.

Promotion The second stage in the multi-stage process of carcinogenesis which must normally follow initiation in order for a tumour to develop.

Psychoactive drugs Drugs which produce behavioural changes.

Ptaquiloside Glucoside of a three ring compound found naturally in bracken which yields a carcinogenic product.

Pulmonary oedema The accumulation of tissue fluid in the air spaces in the lungs.

Quantal response. A response which is all-or-none rather than graded.

Rainout Removal of acids from the atmosphere by rain.

Raynauds phenomenon Changes in the blood supply to the fingers and toes which when caused by vinyl chloride results from degeneration of small blood vessels leading to occlusion of capillaries and arterioles.

Reaginic Relating to reagin, an antibody of the IgE type.

Renal elimination Excretion of a substance through the kidneys.

Rhinitis Inflammation of the mucous membranes of the nose.

Ribosomes The intracellular organelles attached to the endoplasmic reticulum which are involved with protein synthesis.

Risk 'Risk is a measure of the probability that an adverse effect will occur'. This may be absolute risk which is the excess risk due to exposure, or relative risk which is the ratio of risk in the exposed to the unexposed population.

Saturated A term applied to a molecule where all the bonds of the carbon atoms are utilized and there are no double or triple bonds.

Silicosis Damage to the lungs caused by exposure to substances such as silica or coal dust.

Singlet Oxygen Oxygen in the singlet, excited state and therefore highly reactive.

Sinusoids Spaces filled with blood which in the liver are a continuation of the capillaries.

Skink Australian reptile.

Smog The term originally used to describe the combination of *smoke* and *fog* which is now termed reducing smog. Photochemical (oxidant) smog is the result of interaction between the pollution caused mainly by car exhausts and sunlight.

Sub-acute (28 or 90-day) An exposure of duration intermediate between acute and chronic.

Superoxide ($O_{\bar{2}}$) The oxygen molecule with an extra and unpaired electron. It is thus a charged free radical.

Symport Membrane carrier system in which two substances are transported in the same direction.

Synergism/synergistic when toxic effect of a mixture is greater than the sum of the toxicities of the components.

Systemic toxicity Toxicity which affects a system in the organism other than and probably distant from the site of application or exposure.

TD_{50} The dose which is toxic to 50 per cent of the population of organisms exposed to the substance *or* a 50 per cent toxic response in a biological system exposed to the substance.

Teratogen/teratogenicity A substance/property of a substance causing abnormalities in the embryo or foetus when administered to the maternal organism.

Therapeutic index The ratio of ED_{50} to TD_{50}.

Thiol SH or sulphydryl group.

TLV Threshold Limit Value. Upper permissive limits of airborne concentrations of substances.

Tolerance When repeated administration of or dosing with a compound leads to a decrease in the potency in the biological activity of that compound.

Uniport Membrane carrier system in which one substance is transported in the one direction.

Unsaturated A term applied to molecules which contain double or triple carbon-carbon bonds.

Urticaria A vascular reaction of the skin marked by the appearance of weals and which may be caused by direct or indirect exposure to a toxic substance. Also known as hives.

Vascularized When relating to tissue meaning that it is supplied with vessels such as arteries or veins.

Vasculitis Inflammation of the vessels of the vascular system.

Vasodilation/vascular dilatation Dilation of blood vessels.

Veno-occlusive disease A particular type of liver damage where the blood vessels and sinusoids of the liver are damaged so that new vessels grow.

Volume of distribution (V_D) The volume of body fluid in which a compound is apparently distributed when administered to an animal.

Washout Removal of acids from clouds by rain.

Zero order process The rate of the process is independent of the concentration of the substance.

Index

Acceptable Daily Intake (ADI) 15, 146
Accumulation
  and chronic dosing 29,
  of acetaldehyde 15
  of fluid 58
  of cadmium 76, 84
  of lactic acid 134
  reduction by metabolism 37
Acetaldehyde, metabolite of ethanol 15
Acetic acid 136
Acetylation 37, 46, 47, 50, 64, 78
Acetylator phenotype 50,
  and hydralazine 64, 66,
  and aromatic amines 78
Acetylcholinesterase, and
    organophosphorus
    compounds 96,97
Acetyltransferase 50
Acid rain 104, 108, 110
Acidosis 128, 134–136
Aconite 2, 3
Active transport 21–23, 32–34,
  and paraquat 98
Acute toxicity 8, 55, 61, 86, 141–143
Acute toxicity tests 141–143
Additive 6, 14, 83, 85, 86, 89, 146
Adverse drug reactions 69
Aflatoxin 87, 88, 128
African Puff Adder, LD_{50} 127
Air pollution 104–106, 109, 110
Aminolaevulinic acid (ALA) 112, 113
Aminolaevulinic acid dehydrase
    (ALAD) 112, 113
Alcohol abuse 15, 71
Alcohol dehydrogenase 41,
  and ethylene glycol/methanol 135,
  136
Alcohol metabolism 51
Aldehyde dehydrogenase 15, 40, 42
Alkaloids 58, 123, 124

Alkylmercury fungicides 119
Allergy/allergic reactions 56–58, 66,
  74, 84, 86, 127, 146
Aluminium 110
Alveolus/alveolar sac 26, 35, 98
  structure 25
Amanita phalloides 128
Amanitins 128
Ames test 147
Amidases 42, 43
Amides 42, 92
Amino acid conjugation 47
Aminolaevulinic acid 112
Aminolaevulinic acid dehydrase 112
Anaphylaxis 58
Aniline 70, 77, 78, 89
  ionisation in GI tract 23, 26
Animal toxins 125, 126
Antagonism 15
Antibody 86
Antidote 3, 4, 63, 100, 135, 145
Antidotes 3, 4, 63
Antifreeze 135
Antigen 57, 66, 74
Antihypertensive drugs 63, 67
Antiport 22
Aplastic anaemia 41
Aqua Toffana 3
Aromatic amines 35, 40, 44–46, 77,
  78, 92
Arsenic 2, 3
Asbestos 24, 25, 27, 55, 59, 73,
  78–80
Asbestosis 73, 79, 80
Aspergillus flavus 87, 128
Asthma 58, 75, 85, 86, 107, 108
ATPases 127
Atropine 123
AUC 28–30
4-aminobiphenyl 78

Barbiturates 30, 33, 49, 63, 70
Belladonna 123
Benzene 35, 38, 40, 41
Benzidine 77, 78
Benzoic acid 26
Bernard 4, 133
Bhopal 5, 8, 145
Bile duct/canaliculi 33, 35, 78
Biliary 33–35, 49
Binding
  to plasma proteins 30, 33, 70
  of carbon monoxide to
    haemoglobin 56, 107, 133
  of mercury to sulphydryl
    groups 118,
  of ricin 125,
  of phalloidin to plasma proteins 128
  of botulinum toxin 129,
Bioaccumulation 143
Biological factors 48
Biological Oxygen Demand (BOD) 121
Biomagnification 94, 117
Biomarkers 60
Biotransformation 36, 38, 39
Biphenyls 30, 36
Bladder cancer 77, 78, 87, 148
Bleach 8, 131
Blood-brain Barrier 30, 118
Blood flow 21, 22, 25, 26, 35, 57, 58,
  77
BOD 121
Bone marrow 41
Botulinum toxin 13, 57, 87, 123, 129
Botulism 87, 129
Bracken 88, 125
Breast milk 36
Breathing rate 25
British Anti-Lewisite 4
Butter Yellow 84, 85
Butylated hydroxytoluene 84

Cadmium 58, 76, 77, 110
Calcium oxalate 135
Cancer 58, 59, 74, 76–81, 86–88
  and air pollution 106
  skin 111
  throat 125
  alcohol and 136
  safety evaluation and 146–148
Cantharidin 126
Car exhausts 105, 107, 110, 111, 133
Carbon Monoxide 113
  binding to haemoglobin 12, 56
  as a pollutant 104, 105, 107, 110
  poisoning 131, 133–135
Carboxyhaemoglobin 107, 134, 135

Carcinogenicity 56, 59, 87, 141, 143,
  144, 147, 148
Carcinogenicity Tests 144
Carson 1, 91, 145
Castor Oil Plant 125
Cell Membrane 20, 56, 66, 79, 125,
  127
Chemical Oxygen Demand (COD) 121,
  128, 129, 131, 139–148
Chemical factors 48
Chirality 48, 69
Chloroacetaldehyde 76
Chloroethylene oxide 76
Chlorofluorocarbons 111
Cholesterol 19
Cholinesterase 49, 69, 92, 96
Chronic exposure 8, 29, 55
  to insecticides 95–96
  to sulphur dioxide 106
  to carbon monoxide 107
  to cadmium 110
  to lead 113
  to pyrrolizidine alkaloids 124
  to aflatoxin 128
  to alcohol 136
Chronic Toxicity 55, 61, 74, 91, 143,
  147
Chronic Toxicity Tests 143
Cigarettes 51, 76, 107, 111
Cirrhosis 124, 136
Classification 13
Clastogenicity 58
Clean Air Act 103
Clearance 30, 36, 87
Clostridium botulinum 87, 129
COD 121
Coniine 123
Conjugation Reactions 43, 44
Consequences of metabolism 48
Control Limit 80
Copperhead snake 127
Coproporphyrin 112, 113
Curare 4
Cyanide 4, 12, 56, 145
Cycasin 35
Cyclamate 85, 86
Cytisine 123
Cytochrome P450 38–40, 62, 66, 68,
  76
Cytolytic reactions 57

DADPM 77, 78
Daphnia 94, 116, 121, 141, 143
DDD 93
DDE 93–95, 116, 118
DDT 30, 36, 49, 92–96, 115, 116, 118

Dealkylation 40, 41
Death Cap 128
Debrisoquine 50, 57, 58, 67, 68
Delaney Clause 86, 148
Dermatitis 8, 58, 74, 75, 145
Dermis 24
Diamondback Rattlesnake 127
Dieldrin 95, 116
Diethylstilboestrol 35
Digoxin 35
Di-isopropylfluorophosphate 13
Dimethylformamide 51
Dinitrotoluene 49
Dinoflagellates 126
Dioscorides 3
Dioxin 13
Distribution of toxic compounds 28
Disulphiram 15
DNA 58, 76, 78, 125, 147, 148
Dominant Lethal Assay 144
Dosage 10, 13–15, 63, 140–142
Dose-Response 3, 9–16, 141, 142,
  146–148
  relationship, and Paracelsus 3
Drug abuse 71
Drug interactions 69
Drug overdoses 29, 61
Drug toxicity 6, 61–63, 70
Drug(s) 6, 61–68, 131,
  abuse of 71
  interactions and 51, 69–70
  safety evaluation of 139–143
4,4'-Diamino-diphenylmethane 77

E Number 83
Ebers Papyrus 2
Ecotoxicity tests 141
ED_{50} 14
Efron 1
Eggs 115, fish 94, 114,
Eggshells 116, 139
Embryogenesis 59
Enterohepatic recirculation 34, 35
Environmental factors 51, 107
Environmental pollutants 6, 7, 103,
  118
Enzyme induction 70
Epidemiology 104, 148
Epidermis 24, 58, 74
Epoxide hydrolase 43
Epping Jaundice 78, 88
Esters 19
Ethanal 15
Ethanol 21, 33, 42, 135,
  metabolism, 136
Ethylene glycol 36, 37, 56, 135, 136

Eutrophication 114
Excretion 19, 29–37, 49, 112, 113,
  128
Exposure 8–9, 55
  to mixtures 14
  repeated 15
  chronic 29, 91, 107, 110, 111, 128,
    136, 137
  biomarkers of 60, 139
  limits 80–81
  lifetime 84, 143
  dietary 87
Extrapolation 87, 146–148

Facilitated Diffusion 21, 23, 3
Fatty Liver 136
Favism 71
Fibrosis 79, 100
Ficks Law 21
Filtration 21, 32, 106
'First-pass metabolism' 29
Fluoroacetate 100
Fluorocitrate 4, 100
Fog 104, 105
Food
  and absorption from GI tract 26, 27
  contaminants 87–89
Food Additives 5, 6, 8, 15, 42 55,
  83–85, 87, 139, 141, 143
Food Chain 7, 94, 115–117, 119
Food contaminants 85, 87, 128
Formaldehyde 135
Formic Acid 123, 125, 126, 132, 135
Free radicals hydroxyl 98
Fungal toxins 128
Furosemide 34

Gastrointestinal tract
  absorption from, 24, 26–29
  biliary excretion and, 35
  liver metabolism and 38,
  route of exposure 55
  absorption of lead and 111
Genetic factors 47, 50
GLP 145
Gluconeogenesis 136
Glucuronic Acid 44, 45, 47, 62, 78
Glucuronide 49, 50
Glue sniffing 137
Glutathione 34, 45, 46, 62, 63, 70, 71
Glutathione transferases 45
Glucose–6-phosphate dehydrogenase
  deficiency 70
Glycine 47
Good Laboratory Practice (GLP) 145
Gut microflora 34, 35

Haem synthesis 112, 113
Haemangiosarcoma 75
Haemodialysis 100, 135
Haemoglobin 12, 56, 107, 112, 113, 133, 134
Haemolytic anaemia 70, 71, 127
Haemoperfusion 100, 135
Haldane 133–135
Half-life 29, 36, 77
Halogenated solvents 137
Halothane 42, 58, 66, 67
heavy metals 47, 114
Heliotropium 123, 124
Hemlock 3, 123
Henderson Hasselbach Equation 22, 26
Hippocrates 2, 111
HLA Type, DR4 64–66
Honey bee venom 126
Household poisons 6, 7
Hydralazine 41, 47, 50, 51, 58, 63–67
Hydration 43
Hydrazines 46
Hydrocarbons 75, 92, 105–108, 110
Hydrogen peroxide 30, 98, 104, 105
Hydrolysis 42, 43, 49, 69, 92, 96, 97
Hydroxylation 40, 41, 50, 68, 78
Hyperkinetic behaviour 85
Hypersensitivity reactions 58

Idiosyncrasy 70
Immune 57, 60, 66, 76
Immune response 57
Immunological 56, 57, 66, 74, 76, 79
Indocyanine Green 35
Industrial chemicals 6, 8, 58, 73, 74, 76, 139, 141, 143, 145
Industrial diseases 8, 73, 74, 78, 81
Inflammation 55, 58, 74
Intestine 23, 26, 27, 33, 34, 50
Ipomeanol 14
Irritants 74, 106
Irritation 9, 56, 58, 74, 77
Isoenzymes 40, 47
Isoniazid 13, 43, 47, 50
Itai-Itai Disease 110

Kettle Descaler 132
Kidney
  structure and function 32, 33, 37,
  damage to 26, 37, 50, 76–77, 98, 110, 112–113, 118, 128, 135
Killer lymphocytes 66
King Mithridates 3

Laburnam 123

LD$_{50}$ 13, 14, 86, 129, 141, 142
Lead 3 23, 26, 56, 107, 110 111–114,
Lipid peroxidation 98
Lipid solubility 20, 21, 117
Lipophilicity 48
Liver ,
  blood to 28, 38
  damage to 14, 34, 50, 62, 63, 66, 71, 75, 76, 78, 84, 88, 93, 124, 128, 136
  first-pass metabolism and, 29
  bile secretion and, 33,34
  disease and metabolism, 51
London Fog 104
Lungs structure of 25,
  absorption via , 24–27, 31, 111
  excretion via 35,
  damage to, 98–100, 107, 108, 131
Lymphocytes 66

Maimmonides 3
Malaoxon 49, 92, 97
Malathion 41, 49, 92, 96, 97
Margin of safety 14, 81, 148
Maximum Exposure Limit (MEL) 15, 76, 80, 147
Maximum Tolerated Dose (MTD) 147
MEL 15, 76, 80, 147
Mercapturic acid 46
Mercury 30, 47, 91, 92, 115, 117–121
Mescaline 128
Mesothelioma 73, 78–80
Metabolism 19, 36–48
  of drugs, 61–69
  first-pass, 29
  induction by DDT, 95
  saturation of, 31, 84, 86
  factors affecting, 48–51
Metabolism of foreign compounds 36, 38, 47, 95
Metallothionein 76, 77
Methaemoglobinaemia 78
Methanol 135, 136
Methylation 47, 148
Methylazoxymethanol 35
Methylisocyanate 5, 145
Methylmercury 118–120
Microbial toxins 129
Micronucleus test 144
Milk 31, 36, 95, 124
Minamata Disease 117, 119, 120
Mithridatic 3
Mixtures 14, 86, 106, 126, 127
Mojave Rattler 127
Molecular weight 33, 34, 36, 76

Monofluoroacetate 100
Monocrotaline 124
Monooxygenase system 38, 68
MTD 147
Mutagenicity 56, 58–60, 87, 141, 143, 144
Mycotoxins 87
4,4'-Methylene-bis–2-chloroaniline (MBOCA) 77

Naphthalene 46
Natural toxins 6, 7, 123, 126, 129
Necrosis 9, 12, 37, 62, 77, 88, 124, 127, 128
New Substances Regulations 143
Nicander of Colophon 3
Nickel 58, 74, 75
Nicotine 125
Nitrogen oxides 8, 25, 40, 78, 104–108, 110
No Observed Adverse Effect Level (NOAEL) 15, 81, 146, 148
NOAEL 15, 81, 146, 148

Occupational exposure limits 81
Opium 2, 3
Orfila 3
Organomercury 47, 119
Organophosphates/organophosphorus compounds 49, 92, 96–98, 139
Oxalic Acid 36, 135
Oxidation reactions 38, 40, 41
Ozone 105–108, 110, 111

Paracelsus 3, 9
Paracetamol 8, 12, 62–63,
  clearance, 36
  factors affecting toxicity, 51, 70
  metabolism, 48, 62–63
  toxicity, 62–63, 145
Paraquat 8, 97–100, 131
Parathion 25, 74, 96
Particulates 25, 105–108
Passive diffusion 21, 26, 28, 30, 33, 35, 36
Pathological state 48, 51
Pennyroyal Oil 124
Pentobarbital 13, 35
Peroxidases 41, 64
Persistence 7, 93–96, 115, 121, 139, 140
Pesticides 1, 7, 9, 49, 91–100, 103, 114, 116, 121, 140
Peters 4
Phagocytosis 23, 26–28
Phalloidin 128

Phalloin 128
Phallolysin 128
Phase 1 metabolism 37, 38
Phase 2 metabolism 37, 38, 43–45
Phenobarbital 33, 70
Phenyl sulphate 38
Phenylbutazone 70
Phocomelia 69
Phosphodiesterases 127
Phospholipase A 126
Phospholipases 127
Phospholipid 21
Phosphomonoesterases 127
Physico-chemical properties 28, 140
Pinocytosis 21, 23, 26, 28
Plankton 94
Plasma
  clearance, 87
  enzymes, 43, 96
  half-life, 31
  level, 28, 29, 31, 33, 68,98, 100, 136, 141
  pH, 26
  proteins, 26, 30 , 33, 70, 128
Plasma level profile 28
Plasma protein binding 30, 33, 70, 128
PM10 107
Pollution 6, 7, 103–111, 114, 115
Polyamines 98
Polybrominated biphenyls 30
Polychlorinated biphenyls 36
Potency 147
Potentiation 14
Precipitation 108
Precipitin reactions 57
Predisposing factors 65–67
Primaquine 70, 71
Procainamide 44, 47, 50
Procaine 13, 44
Propylbenzene 40
Proteases 77
Protein(s)
  membrane, 19, 21
  plasma, 26, 30, 33, 70, 128
  reactions of compounds with, 30, 57, 60, 62, 66, 76, 88
  excretion and, 32
  denaturation, 74
  as toxins, 125–127
  sulphydryl groups in, 118
Protoporphyrin 112
Psilocin 128
Ptaquiloside 88, 125
Puffer Fish 126, 127
Putrescine 98
Pyrrolizidine alkaloids 123

Quantal   14, 15

Rain out   108
Rapid acetylators   78
Reaginic   57
Receptors   12, 15, 79
Reduction   42, 67, 79, 93, 95, 98, 103, 111, 112
Reproductive toxicity tests   144
Respiratory system   25, 26, 74
Responses   9, 10–15, 56
  detection of, 60
  factors affecting   48–51,
Ribonucleases   127
Ricin   125
Rifampicin   70
Risk Assessment   145, 146, 148, 149
Risk/benefit   91
Route of administration   13, 141, 142
Russels Viper   127

Saccharin   84–87, 147, 148
Salmonella   83
Saturation   19, 29, 33, 34, 84, 107, 134
Saxitoxin   126
Sex   48–50, 64, 66, 71, 140, 142
Silent Spring   1, 91, 145
Silicosis   73
Skin   24–25
  absorption, 24–25, 55, 75, 93, 113
  corrosives and, 7
  diseases, 73–74
  exposure, 8, 140
  irritation, 58
  reactions, 85
  sensitization, 80, 141, 143, 145
  tumours, 59, 111
Skin Absorption   24–25, 55, 75, 93, 113
Slow acetylators   50, 64, 65, 78
Smog   103, 105, 106
Smooth endoplasmic reticulum   38
Snake Venoms   56, 126, 127
Solvents   7, 8, 24–26, 28, 71, 74, 80, 131, 137
Spanish Oil Syndrome   88
Species differences
  in toxicity   13, 78, 91
  pH of GI tract, 26
  as a factor in toxic responses, 48–49
  toxicity testing and, 140, 143, 145, 146, 148
Spermine   98
Strain   49, 50, 143, 148
Succinylcholine   69
Sulphanilamide   46

Sulphate   36, 38, 44, 45, 62, 110
Sulphation   44
Sulphonamides   37, 46
Sulphotransferase   44
Sulphur Dioxide   8, 25, 104–106, 108, 110
Sulphydryl group   45
Superoxide   98, 99
Superoxide dismutase   99
Symport   22
Synergistic   14, 80, 106
Synergistic effect   14, 80, 106

Tartrazine   42, 43, 85, 86
TD_{50} 14
Teratogenicity   58, 141, 143, 144, 147
Testicular toxicity   76, 77, 144
Tetraethyl lead   111, 113
Tetrodotoxin   57, 126, 127
Thalidomide   58, 61, 69
Therapeutic Index   14, 147
Thiopental   30
Threshold dose   15, 147
Threshold limit value (TLV)   15, 76, 80, 147
TLV   15, 76, 80, 147
Tolerance   15, 100
o-Tolidine   78
Toluene   137
Toluene di-isocyanate   58, 75
Total Body Clearance   30
Toxic response   9, 12, 51, 56, 58
Toxic Responses   48, 50, 51, 60, 139
Toxicity tests   76, 121, 139–148
Toxicon   2
Trichloroethane   92, 93, 137
Trifluoroacetylchloride   66
Triglycerides   136
Trp 1   87
Trp 2   87
Type III immune reaction   66

Uniport   22
Uranium dioxide   24, 26, 74
Urinary excretion   32, 49
Urticaria   84–86

V_D 28–30
Vedas   2
Veno-occlusive disease   124
Villi   26
Vinca alkaloids   58
Vinyl chloride   40, 58, 59, 75, 76, 119
Volume of Distribution (V_D)   28

Warfarin   70, 92

Washout 108
Water pollution 114
Wet deposition 110

Whole Body Burden 29

Yellow Card System 140